Diagnosis of Dementia and Cognitive Impairment

Diagnosis of Dementia and Cognitive Impairment

Special Issue Editor

Andrew J. Larner

MDPI • Basel • Beijing • Wuhan • Barcelona • Belgrade

MDPI

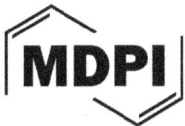

Special Issue Editor
Andrew J. Larner
Walton Centre for Neurology & Neurosurgery
UK

Editorial Office
MDPI
St. Alban-Anlage 66
4052 Basel, Switzerland

This is a reprint of articles from the Special Issue published online in the open access journal *Diagnostics* (ISSN 2075-4418) in 2019 (available at: https://www.mdpi.com/journal/diagnostics/special_issues/dementia_diagnosis).

For citation purposes, cite each article independently as indicated on the article page online and as indicated below:

LastName, A.A.; LastName, B.B.; LastName, C.C. Article Title. *Journal Name* **Year**, *Article Number*, Page Range.

ISBN 978-3-03921-884-4 (Pbk)
ISBN 978-3-03921-885-1 (PDF)

Contents

About the Special Issue Editor

Andrew J. Larner, Consultant Neurologist, is based at the Cognitive Function Clinic, Walton Centre for Neurology and Neurosurgery, Liverpool, UK. He has written and edited a number of books on the subject of dementia and cognitive disorders, based on his experiences working in this area over the past 20 years.

![diagnostics](diagnostics logo) *diagnostics*

MDPI

Editorial

Diagnosis of Dementia and Cognitive Impairment

Andrew J. Larner

Cognitive Function Clinic, Walton Centre for Neurology and Neurosurgery, Lower Lane, Fazakerley, Liverpool L9 7LJ, UK; a.larner@thewaltoncentre.nhs.uk

Received: 31 October 2019; Accepted: 3 November 2019; Published: 7 November 2019

Abstract: In this special issue of *Diagnostics*, expert contributors have produced up-to-date research studies and reviews on various topics related to the diagnosis of dementia and cognitive impairment. The methods of the assessments discussed extend from simple neurological signs, which may be elicited in the clinical encounter, through cognitive screening instruments, to sophisticated analyses of neuroimaging and cerebrospinal fluid biomarkers of disease. It is hoped that these various methods may facilitate earlier diagnosis of dementia and its subtypes, and provide differential diagnosis of depression and functional cognitive disorders, as a prelude to meaningful interventions.

Keywords: dementia; diagnosis; mild cognitive impairment

Dementia and cognitive impairment represent one of the most pressing medical issues of our time, an issue that is likely to escalate as the world population ages. The consequences of this evolving demography pose huge challenges, from the clinical, social, and economic perspectives. Hence, this special issue devoted to the "Diagnosis of Dementia and Cognitive Impairment".

From the clinical standpoint, diagnosis of dementia and cognitive impairment is often the starting point for intervention. The need to identify individuals with dementia and cognitive impairment in order to initiate appropriate treatment and management options is self-evident, yet it remains the case that many afflicted individuals remain undiagnosed, the so-called "dementia diagnosis gap". However, increasing societal awareness of dementia may have prompted an increased frequency of presentation of individuals with purely subjective memory complaints, making functional cognitive disorders an important differential diagnosis of dementia and cognitive impairment.

Various methods to facilitate the accurate diagnosis of dementia and cognitive impairment may be used. These include neurological history taking and clinical examination for particular signs, the administration of cognitive screening instruments, various neuroimaging techniques, and the examination of cerebrospinal fluid for disease biomarkers. All are addressed in this volume.

History taking, both anamnesis, and heteroamnesis, is central to initial patient assessment when either mild cognitive impairment (MCI) or dementia is suspected. This is supplemented by the neurological examination, wherein certain signs may point to the diagnosis. These include both traditional ("canonical") textbook neurological signs and more recently investigated ("non-canonical") signs, such as the attended alone sign, the head-turning sign, and the applause sign [1]. In this issue, Professor Ahmet Turan Isik and his colleagues, who have previously combined these signs as the "Triple Test" [2], show their utility in combination with a cognitive screening instrument, the Rapid Cognitive Screening Test, for the assessment of older adults [3].

Cognitive screening instruments using pencil and paper tests, which are easily applicable at the clinical level, continue to be a mainstay of assessment for cognitive impairment and dementia, particularly in resource-poor or resource-limited settings. There is no shortage of such tests [4], all with their potential advantages and shortcomings. Jerry Brown and his colleagues present an update on the Test Your Memory (TYM) test, which is self-administered under supervision, and the TYM-MCI (formerly Hard-TYM) for the diagnosis of amnestic MCI and mild AD, which is clinician-administered [5]. New data on the use of TYM in a general neurology clinic and as a telephone-administered test are presented, suggesting potential value in these settings [6]. Hartmut Lehfeld and Mark Stemmler demonstrate the potential utility of the Syndrom Kurtztest (SKT), a short cognitive performance test addressing memory and attention, the latter related to the speed of information processing [7]. Ronan O'Caoimh and William Molloy compare the standardised Mini-Mental State Examination (sMMSE) to the Quick Mild Cognitive Impairment (Qmci) screen, finding the latter to have similar or greater accuracy in distinguishing all dementia subtypes and particularly MCI [8]. I present data from a large pragmatic study of the Mini-Addenbrooke's Cognitive Examination (MACE) [9,10], and with Besa Ziso describe attempts to modify the Cognitive Disorders Examination (Codex) [11] to improve detection of MCI [12].

Although routinely and widely used, pencil and paper, cognitive screening tests have many shortcomings. Emma Elliott, Terry Quinn, and their colleagues identify factors associated with full or partial incompletion of cognitive screeners in the context of stroke, finding that around a quarter of patients were fully untestable. The clock drawing test proved the most incomplete of the tests [13]. These issues of test feasibility and how best to handle incomplete data remain to be resolved [14]. Some of the problems with pencil and paper cognitive screening tests might be circumvented by using computerised testing batteries. Reviewing this approach, Avital Sternin, Alistair Burns, and Adrian Owen note advantages such as personalised assessment, at-home testing, measurement of response times, and interpretation of test scores in the context of extensive normative data, permitting the use of "meaningful change" and "validity" indices [15].

Disease biomarkers may be characterised into various subtypes, including diagnostic, predictive, monitoring, and prognostic. Hitherto largely tools of research, biomarkers are now incorporated into diagnostic criteria for neurodegenerative disorders (e.g., Alzheimer's disease [16,17], dementia with Lewy bodies [18]) and their assessment is increasingly becoming part of day-to-day clinical practice. A comprehensive overview of the use of amyloid positron emission tomography (PET) in Alzheimer's disease is provided here by Subapriya Suppiah, Mellanie-Anne Didier, and Sobhan Vinjamuri [19]. Cerebrospinal fluid (CSF) biomarkers have been extensively studied by Miguel Tábuas-Pereira and his colleagues, for example, in connection with the head-turning sign [20] and seizures in Alzheimer's disease [21]. Herein, they suggest a novel potential role for CSF amyloid as a prognostic biomarker for reduced survival in a cohort of patients with frontotemporal dementia [22].

Dementia and cognitive impairment have a broad differential diagnosis [23]. In clinical practice, one of the most challenging differentials is depression, which may be both a risk factor for, and comorbid with, dementia. This interaction is illustrated by O'Caoimh and Molloy, who found that patients with both dementia and depression scored higher on cognitive screening tests (sMMSE and Qmci) than those with dementia only, whereas patients with both MCI and depression scored lower on these tests than those with MCI only. Hence, comorbid depression lowered the diagnostic accuracy of sMMSE and Qmci for dementia, but improved accuracy in those with MCI. O'Caoimh and Molloy suggest that comorbid depression may influence performance on cognitive testing in different ways depending on the stage of cognitive impairment, more so at earlier stages, perhaps increasing the risk of conversion to dementia [8]. Lehfeld and Stemmler show how the subtests of the SKT, examining memory and attention (speed of information processing), may assist in the differential diagnosis of depression versus MCI/mild dementia [7].

Another differential to be considered when assessing patients for dementia and cognitive impairment, and of increasing clinical relevance, is a functional cognitive disorder (FCD) [24]. Catherine Pennington, Harriet Ball, and Marta Swirski report their findings in a series of patients with FCD, noting an equivalent burden of cognitive symptomatology to MCI patients and similar impairment on a cognitive screening instrument (Montreal Cognitive Assessment) [25], as has also been noted with the MACE [26]. Disturbances of mood and sleep may be contributory factors to FCD [26]. Using the large datasets generated by online testing, Sternin, Burns, and Owen note that whilst older people sleep less, the amount of sleep required for optimal cognitive performance remains constant regardless of age, suggesting that more sleep may be a good idea as we age [15].

As this brief overview shows, the primary aims of this special issue have been to present information on promising new approaches to diagnose dementia and cognitive impairment, which are readily applicable to clinical practice and which also assist in the significant differential diagnosis of functional cognitive disorders. But what of the future? The dismal outcomes of clinical therapeutic trials for Alzheimer's disease in recent years (which contrast so starkly with the great increase in understanding of the biology of the disease [27]) have suggested that by the time of clinical diagnosis the degree of brain injury may be largely irreversible, thereby demanding a proactive preventative approach to maintain brain health rather than a reactive therapeutic response to palliate brain disease. How might the preclinical, presymptomatic phases of the disease, which are recognised to be of decades duration [28], be reliably and accurately identified, and hence amenable to the application of (yet to be identified) disease-modifying treatments?

One way forward may be suggested by a recent report finding accelerated long term forgetting to be a feature of presymptomatic stages of (autosomal dominant) Alzheimer's disease [29]. Obviously, the finding requires independent corroboration, but if true, it might indicate one approach to the "bioprediction" of Alzheimer's disease, perhaps in combination with amyloid PET imaging and CSF biomarkers and genetic panels examining risk factor alleles. The bioprediction approach seeks to conceptualise medical "disorder" in terms of probabilistic modelling, based on present and future risks of harm rather on a binary or categorical formulation (disorder or normalcy) and is justified by the belief that disease biomarkers will not map cleanly onto clinical diagnostic categories. "Risk banding", based on the shape of a "probability dysfunction" model unique to each individual, might be used to determine the necessity or otherwise for response/intervention [30].

It has been a great honor and privilege for me to guest edit this timely special issue. I am grateful to all the authors for their willingness to contribute and for their prompt submission of manuscripts. I hope readers will derive as much interest and stimulus in reading these articles as I have in curating them.

Conflicts of Interest: The author declares no conflict of interest.

References

1. Larner, A.J. Neurological signs of possible diagnostic value in the cognitive disorders clinic. *Pract. Neurol.* **2014**, *14*, 332–335. [CrossRef] [PubMed]
2. Isik, A.T.; Soysal, P.; Kaya, D.; Usarel, C. Triple test, a diagnostic observation, can detect cognitive impairment in older adults. *Psychogeriatrics* **2018**, *18*, 98–105. [CrossRef] [PubMed]
3. Okudur, S.K.; Dokuzlar, O.; Kaya, D.; Soysal, P.; Isik, A.T. Triple Test plus Rapid Cognitive Screening Test: a combination of clinical signs and a tool for cognitive assessment in older adults. *Diagnostics* **2019**, *9*, 97. [CrossRef] [PubMed]
4. Larner, A.J. (Ed.) *Cognitive Screening Instruments. A Practical Approach*, 2nd ed.; Springer: London, UK, 2017. [CrossRef]
5. Brown, J.M. TYM (Test Your Memory) testing. In *Cognitive Screening Instruments. A Practical Approach*, 2nd ed.; Larner, A.J., Ed.; Springer: London, UK, 2017; pp. 209–229. [CrossRef]
6. Brown, J.M.; Wiggins, J.; Dawson, K.; Rittman, T.; Rowe, J.B. Test Your Memory (TYM) and Test Your Memory for Mild Cognitive Impairment (TYM-MCI): A review and update including results of using the TYM Test in a general neurology clinic and using a telephone version of the TYM Test. *Diagnostics* **2019**, *9*, 116. [CrossRef] [PubMed]
7. Lehfeld, H.; Stemmler, S. The newly normed SKT reveals differences in neuropsychological profiles of patients with MCI, mild dementia and depression. *Diagnostics* **2019**, *9*, 163. [CrossRef]
8. O'Caoimh, R.; Molloy, D.W. Comparing the diagnostic accuracy of two cognitive screening instruments in different dementia subtypes and clinical depression. *Diagnostics* **2019**, *9*, 93. [CrossRef]

9. Hsieh, S.; McGrory, S.; Leslie, F.; Dawson, K.; Ahmed, S.; Butler, C.R.; Rowe, J.B.; Mioshi, E.; Hodges, J.R. The Mini-Addenbrooke's Cognitive Examination: A new assessment tool for dementia. *Dement. Geriatr. Cogn. Disord.* **2015**, *39*, 1–11. [CrossRef]

10. Larner, A.J. MACE for diagnosis of dementia and MCI: examining cut-offs and predictive values. *Diagnostics* **2019**, *9*, 51. [CrossRef]

11. Belmin, J.; Pariel-Madjlessi, S.; Surun, P.; Bentot, C.; Feteanu, D.; des Noettes, V.L.; Onen, F.; Drunat, O.; Trivalle, C.; Chassagne, P.; et al. The cognitive disorders examination (Codex) is a reliable 3-min test for detection of dementia in the elderly (validation study in 323 subjects). *Presse Med.* **2007**, *36*, 1183–1190.

12. Ziso, B.; Larner, A.J. Codex (Cognitive Disorders Examination) decision tree modified for the detection of dementia and MCI. *Diagnostics* **2019**, *9*, 58. [CrossRef]

13. Elliott, E.; Drozdowska, B.A.; Taylor-Rowan, M.; Shaw, R.C.; Cuthbertson, G.; Quinn, T.J. Who is classified as untestable on brief cognitive screens in an acute stroke setting? *Diagnostics* **2019**, *9*, 95. [CrossRef] [PubMed]

14. Lees, R.A.; Hendry, B.K.; Broomfield, N.; Stott, D.; Larner, A.J.; Quinn, T.J. Cognitive assessment in stroke: feasibility and test properties using differing approaches to scoring of incomplete items. *Int. J. Geriatr. Psychiatry* **2017**, *32*, 1072–1078. [CrossRef] [PubMed]

15. Sternin, A.; Burns, A.; Owen, A.M. Thirty-five years of computerized cognitive assessment of aging—where are we now? *Diagnostics* **2019**, *9*, 114. [CrossRef] [PubMed]

16. Albert, M.S.; DeKosky, S.T.; Dickson, D.; Dubois, B.; Feldman, H.H.; Fox, N.C.; Gamst, A.; Holtzman, D.M.; Jagust, W.J.; Petersen, R.C.; et al. The diagnosis of mild cognitive impairment due to Alzheimer's disease: Recommendations from the National Institute on Aging-Alzheimer's Association workgroups on diagnostic guidelines for Alzheimer's disease. *Alzheimers Dement.* **2011**, *7*, 270–279. [CrossRef]

17. Dubois, B.; Feldman, H.H.; Jacova, C.; Hampel, H.; Molinuevo, J.L.; Blennow, K.; DeKosky, S.T.; Gauthier, S.; Selkoe, D.; Bateman, R.; et al. Advancing research diagnostic criteria for Alzheimer's disease: The IWG-2 criteria. *Lancet Neurol.* **2014**, *13*, 614–629. [CrossRef]

18. McKeith, I.G.; Boeve, B.F.; Dickson, D.W.; Halliday, G.; Taylor, J.P.; Weintraub, D.; Aarsland, D.; Galvin, J.; Attems, J.; Ballard, C.G.; et al. Diagnosis and management of dementia with Lewy bodies: Fourth consensus report of the DLB Consortium. *Neurology* **2017**, *89*, 88–100. [CrossRef]

19. Suppiah, S.; Didier, M.A.; Vinjamuri, S. The who, when, why, and how of PET amyloid imaging in management of Alzheimer's disease—Review of literature and interesting images. *Diagnostics* **2019**, *9*, 65. [CrossRef]

20. Durães, J.; Tábuas-Pereira, M.; Araujo, R.; Duro, D.; Baldeiras, I.; Santiago, B.; Santana, I. The head turning sign in dementia and mild cognitive impairment: its relationship to cognition, behavior, and cerebrospinal fluid markers. *Dement. Geriatr. Cogn. Disord.* **2018**, *46*, 42–49. [CrossRef]

21. Tábuas-Pereira, M.; Durães, J.; Lopes, J.; Sales, F.; Bento, C.; Duro, D.; Santiago, B.; Almeida, M.R.; Leitão, M.J.; Baldeiras, I.; et al. Increased CSF tau is associated with a higher risk of seizures in patients with Alzheimer's disease. *Epilepsy Behav.* **2019**, *98*, 207–209. [CrossRef]

22. Vieira, D.; Durães, J.; Baldeiras, I.; Santiago, B.; Duro, D.; Lima, M.; Leitão, M.J.; Tábuas-Pereira, M.; Santana, I. Lower CSF amyloid-beta1–42 predicts a higher mortality rate in frontotemporal dementia. *Diagnostics* **2019**, *9*, 162. [CrossRef]

23. Larner, A.J. *Neuropsychological Neurology: The Neurocognitive Impairments of Neurological Disorders*, 2nd ed.; Cambridge University Press: Cambridge, UK, 2013. [CrossRef]

24. Stone, J.; Pal, S.; Blackburn, D.; Reuber, M.; Thekkumpurath, P.; Carson, A. Functional (psychogenic) cognitive disorders: A perspective from the neurology clinic. *J. Alzheimers Dis.* **2015**, *48* (Suppl. 1), S5–S17. [CrossRef] [PubMed]

25. Pennington, C.; Ball, H.; Swirski, M. Functional cognitive disorder: diagnostic challenges and future directions. *Diagnostics* **2019**, *9*, 131. [CrossRef] [PubMed]

26. Bharambe, V.; Larner, A.J. Functional cognitive disorders: demographic and clinical features contribute to a positive diagnosis. *Neurodegener. Dis. Manag.* **2018**, *8*, 377–383. [CrossRef] [PubMed]

27. Macreadie, I. (Ed.) *Molecular mechanism of Alzheimer's Disease*; MDPI: Basel, Switzerland, 2019.

28. Jack, C.R., Jr.; Knopman, D.S.; Jagust, W.J.; Petersen, R.C.; Weiner, M.W.; Aisen, P.S.; Shaw, L.M.; Vemuri, P.; Wiste, H.J.; Weigand, S.D.; et al. Tracking pathophysiological processes in Alzheimer's disease: An updated hypothetical model of dynamic biomarkers. *Lancet Neurol.* **2013**, *12*, 207–216. [CrossRef]

Diagnostics **2019**, *9*, 180

29. Weston, P.S.J.; Nicholas, J.M.; Henley, S.M.D.; Liang, Y.; Macpherson, K.; Donnachie, E.; Schott, J.M.; Rossor, M.N.; Crutch, S.J.; Butler, C.R.; et al. Accelerated long-term forgetting in presymptomatic autosomal dominant Alzheimer's disease: A cross-sectional study. *Lancet Neurol.* **2018**, *17*, 123–132. [CrossRef]

30. Baum, M.L. *The Neuroethics of Biomarkers. What the Development of Bioprediction Means for Moral Responsibility, Justice, and the Nature of Mental Disorder*; Oxford University Press: Oxford, UK, 2016.

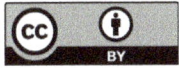

diagnostics

MDPI

Article

Triple Test Plus Rapid Cognitive Screening Test: A Combination of Clinical Signs and A Tool for Cognitive Assessment in Older Adults

Saadet Koc Okudur [1], Ozge Dokuzlar [2], Derya Kaya [2], Pinar Soysal [3] and Ahmet Turan Isik [2,*]

[1] Department of Geriatric Medicine, Manisa State Hospital, Manisa 45040, Turkey
[2] Unit for Brain Aging and Dementia, Department of Geriatric Medicine, Faculty of Medicine, Dokuz Eylul University, Izmir 35340, Turkey
[3] Department of Geriatric Medicine, Faculty of Medicine, Bezmialem Vakif University, Istanbul 34093, Turkey
* Correspondence: atisik@yahoo.com; Tel.: +90-232-412-43-41

Received: 29 June 2019; Accepted: 13 August 2019; Published: 15 August 2019

Abstract: Less time-consuming, easy-to-apply and more reliable cognitive screening tests are essential for use in primary care. The aim of this study was to investigate the diagnostic value of the Turkish version of the Rapid Cognitive Screen (RCS-T) and Triple Test individually and the combination of RCS-T with each sign and Triple Test to screen elderly patients for cognitive impairment (CI). A total of 357 outpatients aged 60 or older, who underwent comprehensive geriatric assessment, were included in the study. Presence or absence of attended alone sign (AAS), head-turning sign, and applause sign was investigated. The mean age of the patients was 74.29 ± 7.46. Of those, 61 patients (28 men, 33 women) had Alzheimer's disease (AD), 59 patients had mild cognitive impairment (MCI) (29 men, 30 women), and 237 (80 men, 157 women) were cognitively robust. The sensitivity of the combination of RCS-T and negative for AAS for CI, AD and MCI is 0.79, 0.86 and 0.61, respectively; the specificity was 0.92, 0.93 and 0.92, respectively; and the positive and negative predictive values revealed good diagnostic accuracy. The combination of RCS-T and negative for AAS is a simple, effective and rapid way to identify possible CI in older adults.

Keywords: cognitive screening instruments; dementia; mild cognitive impairment; cognitive impairment; Rapid Cognitive Screen; Triple Test

---

1. Introduction

Memory complaints, which should be distinguished from cognitive impairments (CI) related to neurodegenerative diseases such as Alzheimer's disease (AD), are quite prevalent among older adults [1,2]. It is difficult to devote time for detailed neuropsychological tests during a busy clinical day, which is the first approach to determine whether or not a patient requires further clinical evaluation for CI [3]. Therefore, less time-consuming, easy-to-apply and more reliable cognitive screening tests (which are essential to accurately diagnose patients with CI, especially for primary care settings) may help primary care professionals determine whether it is necessary to refer a patient to a tertiary care or a memory center for cognitive diseases [4].

Elaborate medical history, physical examination, and neurocognitive assessment should be performed to identify the etiology of memory loss [5]. The Rapid Cognitive Screen (RCS) is a brief screening tool derived from the Saint Louis University Mental Status (SLUMS) examination for the detection of cognitive dysfunction in primary care settings [6] and the Turkish version of the RCS (RCS-T) is validated in Turkish older adults [7]. Additionally, inclusion of some clinical signs of neurodegenerative diseases leading to dementia, such as the attended alone sign (AAS) [8], head-turning sign (HTS) [9,10] and applause sign (AS) [11] in cognitive assessment, may play a significant role in the diagnostic process [4,12].

The Triple Test consisting of AAS, HTS and AS has been shown to be a simple, rapid and effective screening tool for detecting cognitive impairment, and deterioration of daily living activities in older adults [4,12]. AS is also called the clapping test, three-clap test, or signe d'applause. The evaluation is as follows: The patient is asked to clap three times as quickly as possible after the examiner had performed a demonstration. When the patient claps three times, this is considered negative for AS. When the patient claps more than three times, this is considered positive for AS. Patients clapping less than three times are considered pathologic, and positive for AS, as reported previously [13,14]. In the literature [9,15], HTS is assessed while the patient's caregiver sat silently at a 45° angle, approximately 1 m behind the patient, who is encouraged to speak about their cognitive function history. When the patient turns her/his head away from the collocutor and towards the caregiver(s) for help, the patient is considered positive for HTS. When the patient did not want any help, this is considered negative for HTS. AAS is evaluated based on whether the patient attended the clinic with a family member, caregiver, or friend. When the patient is accompanied, this is considered negative for attended alone sign [15].

Early definitive diagnosis of cognitive impairment may be difficult in busy clinic settings, in which the main purpose of combining tests is to ensure early recognition of patients with cognitive impairment and referral to a higher center.

Nevertheless, it is not known whether the combination of the RCS-T test, a clinical screening tool, and the Triple Test, a test based on clinical symptoms, has positive effects on the management of memory problems. Therefore, in the present study we aimed to investigate the diagnostic value of the RCS-T and Triple Test individually and the combination of RCS-T with each sign and Triple Test to screen elderly patients for CI.

2. Materials and Methods

A total of 357 patients aged over 60 years, who were admitted to the geriatric outpatient clinic with memory complaints between June 2014 and February 2019, and underwent comprehensive geriatric assessment, were included in the study. All the participants, who provided informed consent to participate in the study, were evaluated by comprehensive geriatric assessment, including physical and mental status examination and laboratory evaluation. The ethics committee of Dokuz Eylul University, Turkey, approved the study protocol with decision number 2018/22-19, and the project identification code is 4241-GOA (September 13, 2018). Each participant or a legal guardian provided written, informed consent to participate in the study. We carried out this study in accordance with the provisions of the Declaration of Helsinki.

Major and minor CI was diagnosed according to the Diagnostic and Statistical Manual of Mental Disorders (fifth edition) diagnostic criteria [16] and AD was diagnosed according to National Institute on Aging–Alzheimer's Association workgroup's criteria [17]. The cognitively robust group consisted of patients who had memory complaints despite normal cognitive assessments and those who attended our geriatric outpatient clinic for prevention programs because of other medical issues.

Socio-demographic characteristics of the patients, including gender, age and education, were recorded. All patients were examined to see if they had hearing loss, cataracts, hypertension, diabetes mellitus, coronary artery disease, peripheral vascular disease, hyperlipidemia, cerebrovascular disease, congestive heart failure, depression, dementia, or polypharmacy in their medical history. For each patient, a comprehensive geriatric assessment, including detailed and complete physical and mental examinations, was performed [18]. Patients were evaluated based on the RCS-T [7], Mini-Mental State Examination (MMSE) [19], Geriatric Depression Scale [20], Instrumental Activities of Daily Living [21], Basic Activities of Daily Living Scale [22], Clinical Dementia Rating, and a clock drawing test. For the patients with CI, further evaluations, such as laboratory examination and brain imaging (essential for the differential diagnosis CI) were also performed.

The signs were assessed by two physicians (S.K.O and O.D.), who were blinded to the diagnosis of the patients. High interrater agreements were observed (1.00 for AAS, 0.98 for HTS, and 1.00 for AS). Presence or absence of AS, AAS, and HTS was investigated.

The RCS test includes 3 items: recall of 5 words, a clock drawing test, and the ability to remember a story [6]. Scores ranged from 0 and 10. The RCS-T optimal cut-off scores were ≤ 4 for dementia and ≤ 6 for mild cognitive impairment (MCI) [7].

Patients with unilateral hearing impairment or blindness and deafness, and those considered to be too sick to be questioned, including those in delirium, were excluded. Those who had been taking medications that might influence their thinking or memory, who had previous head trauma resulting in unconsciousness and/or a period of memory impairment, who were unable to provide informed consent to participate in the study, who cannot speak Turkish, or who were illiterate, were excluded. Reversible CI related to vitamin B12 or folic acid deficiency, hypothyroidism, subdural hematoma, hyponatremia, medications (e.g., corticosteroids, antipsychotics, and benzodiazepines), substance abuse problems and the institutionalized older adults were excluded.

The package program, Statistical Package for Social Sciences (SPSS) version 23.0 for Windows (SPSS Inc., Chicago, IL, USA), was used for the statistical analysis. Descriptive statistics are presented as means ± standard deviations or percentages. Nominal variables were evaluated by Pearson's χ2-test. Kruskal–Wallis test was used to analyze the presence of non-normal distribution, and continuous variables with normal distribution were assessed with one-way ANOVA (shown as the P_1 value in Table 1). Adjustment according to age and gender was carried out by multinomial logistic regression analysis (shown as the P_2 and P_3 value in Table 1). Sensitivity refers to proportion of correct positive classifications, and specificity refers to proportion of correct negative classifications. p-value < 0.05 was considered significant. Sensitivity, specificity, and positive and negative predictive values (PPV, NPV) were calculated for diagnosis of any CI, AD, and MCI. A sample size of 214 participants was calculated as the minimum required size to be within a 5% of the true proportion.

Table 1. Descriptive characteristics of participants ($n = 357$).

	Control ($n = 237$)	MCI ($n = 59$)	AD ($n = 61$)	P_1	P_2	P_3
Women (%)	66.2	51.7	53.3	0.041	-	-
Age	72.45 ± 7.08	76.37 ± 6.09	78.95 ± 7.63	<0.001	-	-
Education (year)	8.61 ± 3.84	7.98 ± 3.76	8.48 ± 4.09	0.390	-	-
Number of drugs	5.33 ± 3.33	5.65 ± 3.02	5.92 ± 3.07	0.214	-	-
MMSE	28.26 ± 1.71	25.25 ± 3.44	17.92 ± 4.86	<0.001	<0.001	<0.001
SLUMS	25.14 ± 3.19	19.50 ± 4.56	10.88 ± 4.64	<0.001	<0.001	<0.001
RCS-T	8.28 ± 1.52	5.42 ± 2.13	2.15	<0.001	<0.001	<0.001
CDR	0.0 ± 0.1	0.5 ± 0.2	1.5 ± 0.6	<0.001	<0.001	<0.001
CDT	4.7 ± 0.8	4.2 ± 1.2	2.2 ± 1.3	<0.001	<0.001	<0.001
GDS	2.8 ± 3.3	3.1 ± 3.3	3.7 ± 3.3	0.139	-	-
BADL	95.46 ± 5.87	93.15 ± 13.22	83.58 ± 18.28	<0.001	<0.001	0.259
IADL	14.99 ± 3.13	13.58 ± 3.94	8.07 ± 4.95	<0.001	<0.001	0.169

AD, Alzheimer's disease; BADL, Basic Activities of Daily Living; CDR, Clinical Dementia Rating; CDT, clock-drawing; GDS, Geriatric Depression Scale; IADL, Instrumental Activities of Daily Living; MCI, mild cognitive impairment; MMSE, Mini-Mental State Examination; P_1, p-values for comparison of three groups; P_2, p-values for comparison of AD and control group after adjusted for age and gender; P_3, p-values for comparison of MCI and control group after adjusted for age and gender; RCS-T, Turkish version of the Rapid Cognitive Screen test; SLUMS, Saint Louis University Mental Status Examination. Score range for each of the assessments: BADL, 0 (worst)–100 (best); CDR, 0 (best)–3 (worst); CDT, 0 (worst)–5 (best); GDS, 0 (best)–15 (worst); IADL, 0 (worst)–17 (best); MMSE, 0 (worst)–30 (best), RCS-T, 0 (worst)–10 (best); SLUMS, 0 (worst)–30 (best). All data are expressed as means ± standard deviations.

3. Results

A total of 357 outpatients (137 men, 220 women) with a mean age of 74.29 ± 7.46 years were assessed. Of the patients, 61 (28 men, 33 women) were diagnosed with AD, 59 were diagnosed with MCI (29 men, 30 women) and 237 (80 men, 157 women) were cognitively robust (controls). There was a significant difference among AD, MCI and controls in terms of gender and age; there were more female participants in controls ($p < 0.05$) and older patients in AD group ($p < 0.001$). There was no difference in the patients with MCI, AD, and controls with regards to total years of education or educational level of the participants (for each, $p > 0.05$). There was no difference for the number of drugs between the groups ($p > 0.05$). After comprehensive geriatric assessment, when MMSE, SLUMS, RCS-T, clinical dementia rating test, clock-drawing test, Geriatric Depression Scale, Basic Activities of Daily Living Scales and Instrumental Activities of Daily Living were evaluated, there was a significant difference between the groups ($p < 0.001$) except for Geriatric Depression Scale. Descriptive data of the patients are summarized in Table 1. After adjustments for age and gender by multinomial logistic regression analysis MMSE, RCS-T, SLUMS, clock-drawing test (CDT), Clinical Dementia Rating (CDR), Basic Activities of Daily Living (BADL), and Instrumental Activities of Daily Living (IADL) were still significant in the AD group compared to the control group ($p < 0.001$). When MCI and control group were compared, statistical significance was maintained for MMSE, SLUMS, RCS-T, CDR, CDT ($p < 0.001$); but BADL ($p = 0.259$) and IADL ($p = 0.169$) showed no statistical significance.

Patients' neuropsychological profiles were assessed based on the presence or absence of AS, HTS and AAS and the neuropsychological tests (MMSE, SLUMS, RCS-T and clock-drawing test). The sensitivity and specificity, and PPV and NPV values of the tests are shown in Table 2.

Table 2. Assessment of the diagnostic value of the RCS-T and Triple Test individually and the combination of RCS-T with each sign and Triple Test.

	Each Test		Combinations of RCS + Each Sign			Combinations of RCS + Triple Test	
	RCS-T	Triple	RCS-T and PHTS	RCS-T and PAS	RCS-T and NAAS	RCS-T and Triple	RCS-T or Triple
CI							
Sensitivity %	85.83	29.66	58.47	29.66	79.66	29.17	86.44
Specificity %	88.19	96.51	96.94	98.69	92.14	98.7	85.59
PPV %	78.63	81.40	90.79	92.11	83.93	92.11	75.56
NPV %	92.48	72.70	81.92	73.14	89.79	72.76	92.45
AD							
Sensitivity %	86.67	42.37	69.49	40.48	86.44	39.49	88.33
Specificity %	90.91	93.75	94.77	98.61	93.03	98.89	85.76
PPV %	65.82	58.14	73.21	85.71	71.83	86.82	56.38
NPV %	97.12	88.82	93.79	88.73	97.09	87.06	97.24
MCI							
Sensitivity %	73.33	15.52	78.79	16.95	61.02	15.25	61.54
Specificity %	88.19	96.51	87.06	98.69	92.14	99.13	87.11
PPV %	61.11	52.94	44.07	76.92	66.67	81.82	45.28
NPV %	92.89	81.85	96.94	82.18	90.17	81.95	92.89

AD, Alzheimer's disease; CI, Cognitive impairment; MCI, Mild cognitive impairment; NAAS, Negative for attended alone sign; NPV, Negative predictive value; PAS, Positive for applause sign; PHTS, Positive for head-turning sign; PPV, Positive predictive value; RCS, Rapid Cognitive Screen test.

4. Discussion

The present study demonstrated that RCS-T and the Triple Test are easy to perform together and are highly specific tools to screen elderly patients with CI, AD or MCI while the combination of RCS-T and negative for AAS is sensitive and specific enough to accurately screen those with CI.

Discrimination between cognitively normal and CI in older adults, especially in early stage, requires long, time-consuming cognitive tests and sophisticated evaluations. For this purpose, many tests are currently available for cognitive screening. Out of them, the sensitivity and specificity of MMSE, Montreal cognitive assessment, Turkish version of SLUMS, and Cognitive state test screening tests are 0.91 and 0.95; 0.81 and 0.78; 0.84 and 0.87; and 0.81 and 0.78, respectively [19,23–25]; however, they tend to be time consuming and may be inappropriate for both bedside clinical evaluation and daily clinical practice, especially in the primary care setting. In a recent study, SLUMS-derived RCS [6,7] has been reported to be a simple, fast and practical tool that is sensitive and specific enough to screen CI in older adults and reflects deterioration in daily living activities [7] which is confirmed once again in the present study.

In addition, it is highly important that physicians consider cognitive screening tools as well as the early clinical signs of specific neurodegenerative diseases, such as HTS, AAS, and AS in order to make a differential diagnosis. The neuropsychological properties of HTS are potentially heterogeneous, including amnesia, impaired comprehension and lack of insight [10]. Previous studies showed that AAS is effective in detecting cognitively robust patients [12,26]. AAS is also thought to give information about instrumental activities of daily living and noncognitive functions in the same domain such as mobility, gait, balance and vision [4,27]. AS is a motor perseveration indicative of frontal lobe dysfunction in different types of dementia [28]. In a recent study, the combination called the Triple Test has been demonstrated to be a simple, quick and efficient screening tool for detecting CI [4].

The present study showed that the combination of RCS-T or the Triple Test positivity has a good sensitivity for discriminating between patients with CI, AD, and MCI (0.86, 0.88 and 0.62, respectively) and also better with higher NPV for all (0.92, 0.97 and 0.93, respectively). It means that the combination can correctly identify older patients without CI among those with memory problems, and that it can be used for older adults with memory complaints in bedside evaluation or primary care setting. Hence, those who are negative for the combination may not need to be referred to the relevant memory centers for detailed cognitive assessment. Additionally, in the present study, RCS-T plus AAS has good sensitivity and high specificity to detect CI in older adults.

When the current results were compared with our previous ones [4], it was found that sensitivity and specificity of the Triple Test were not similar in these studies, which can be explained by gender and educational differences, considering the fact that some cultural and methodological differences should be kept in mind while assessing the results of the studies [29].

Of particular note in this study, the RCS-T test together with HTS showed a remarkable NPV (0.97), which may be a signal or alert to closely monitor individuals with the possibility of MCI or to refer to the memory centers. With this finding, using RCS-T and positive for HTS together can be considered as a daily questionnaire because the RCS-T test is a reliable and valid measure, and indeed doctors inevitably evaluate HTS during routine history taking. Unfortunately, there is no specific applicable measurement to differentiate those with MCI from those that are cognitively robust, but measurements are increasingly being investigated for early detection of AD/MCI. Recently, it has been shown that Addenbrooke's Cognitive Examination III has a sensitivity of 0.77 and specificity 0.92 in capturing individuals with MCI in Japan [30], and a sensitivity of 0.63 and specificity of 0.63 in Malay [31]. Our finding, with a sensitivity of 0.78 and specificity of 0.87, is also compatible with the aforementioned studies.

RCS-T alone is also very valuable due to the fact that it differentiated cognitively robust older adults accurately from those who had MCI or cognitive impairment. In the present study, RCS-T is combined with Triple Test, which is performed by physicians during the physical examination. It is striking that specificity of the combination was high enough to show that individuals with a good test performance are healthy. Furthermore, patients who have poor performance for either RCS-T or Triple Test are more likely to be cognitively impaired, with a sensitivity of 0.86. Therefore, older people with memory problems could be better directed for further neurocognitive analysis if either of them is positive.

The strengths of this study are the large sample size and that all the cases included in the study were over 60 years of age. As far as we are concerned, this is the first study to evaluate the diagnostic value of the combination; however, it has still some limitations. Since it was conducted at a memory center, the generalizability of our findings might be limited. Another limitation is that HTS requires the presence of a person accompanying the patient to the clinic.

5. Conclusions

Our study has demonstrated that the combination of RCS-T and negative for AAS is simple, effective and rapid way to identify possible CI in older adults. The combination of RCS-T and Triple Test has the ability to identify the cognitively robust older adults with subjective memory complaints, while those with poor performance for either of them may require further neurocognitive evaluation for CI. Therefore, the combination of both tests could serve as an indicator of those patients in need of further neurocognitive analysis, especially in daily busy clinical practice.

Author Contributions: Conceptualization, P.S. and A.T.I.; formal analysis, O.D.; investigation, S.K.O. and D.K.; methodology, A.T.I.; writing—review & editing, S.K.O., P.S. and A.T.I.

Funding: This research received no external funding.

Conflicts of Interest: The authors declare no conflict of interest.

References

1. Ates Bulut, E.; Soysal, P.; Yavuz, I.; Kocyigit, S.E.; Isik, A.T. Effect of Vitamin D on Cognitive Functions in Older Adults: 24-Week Follow-Up Study. *Am. J. Alzheimers Dis. Other Demen* **2019**, *34*, 112–117. [CrossRef] [PubMed]
2. Reitz, C.; Brayne, C.; Mayeux, R. Epidemiology of Alzheimer disease. *Nat. Rev. Neurol.* **2011**, *7*, 137–152. [CrossRef] [PubMed]
3. Cordell, C.B.; Borson, S.; Boustani, M.; Chodosh, J.; Reuben, D.; Verghese, J.; Thies, W.; Fried, L.B. Alzheimer's Association recommendations for operationalizing the detection of cognitive impairment during the Medicare Annual Wellness Visit in a primary care setting. *Alzheimers Dement.* **2013**, *9*, 141–150. [CrossRef] [PubMed]
4. Isik, A.T.; Soysal, P.; Kaya, D.; Usarel, C. Triple test, a diagnostic observation, can detect cognitive impairment in older adults. *Psychogeriatrics* **2018**, *18*, 98–105. [CrossRef] [PubMed]
5. Annoni, J.; Chouiter, L.; Demonet, J. Age-related cognitive impairment: Conceptual changes and diagnostic strategies. *Rev. Méd. Suisse* **2016**, *12*, 774–779. [PubMed]
6. Malmstrom, T.K.; Voss, V.B.; Cruz-Oliver, D.M.; Cummings-Vaughn, L.A.; Tumosa, N.; Grossberg, G.T.; Morley, J.E. The Rapid Cognitive Screen (RCS): A point-ofcare screening for dementia and mild cognitive impairment. *J. Nutr. Health Aging* **2015**, *19*, 741–744. [CrossRef]
7. Koc Okudur, S.; Dokuzlar, O.; Usarel, C.; Soysal, P.; Isik, A.T. Validity and Reliability of Rapid Cognitive Screening Test for Turkish Older Adults. *J. Nutr. Health Aging* **2019**, *23*, 68–72. [CrossRef]
8. Larner, A.J. 'Who came with you?' A diagnostic observation in patients with memory problems? *J. Neurol. Neurosurg. Psychiatry* **2005**, *76*, 1739. [CrossRef]
9. Fukui, T.; Yamazaki, T.; Kinno, R. Can the 'head-turning sign' be a clinical marker of Alzheimer's disease? *Dement. Geriatr. Cogn. Disord. Extra* **2011**, *1*, 310–317. [CrossRef]
10. Larner, A.J. Head turning sign: Pragmatic utility in clinical diagnosis of cognitive impairment. *J. Neurol. Neurosurg. Psychiatry* **2012**, *83*, 852–853. [CrossRef]
11. Dubois, B.; Slachevsky, A.; Pillon, B.; Beato, R.; Villalponda, J.M.; Liyvan, I. 'Applause sign' helps to discriminate PSP from FTD and PD. *Neurology* **2005**, *64*, 2132–2133. [CrossRef] [PubMed]
12. Soysal, P.; Usarel, C.; Ispirli, G.; Isik, A.T. Attended with and headturning sign can be clinical markers of cognitive impairment in older adults. *Int. Psychogeriatr.* **2017**, *29*, 1–7. [CrossRef] [PubMed]

13. Wu, L.J.; Sitburana, O.; Davidson, A.; Jankovic, J. Applause sign in Parkinsonian disorders and Huntington's disease. *Mov. Disord.* **2008**, *23*, 2307–2311. [CrossRef] [PubMed]
14. Isella, V.; Rucci, F.; Traficante, D.; Mapelli, C.; Ferri, F.; Appollonio, I.M. The applause sign in cortical and cortical-subcortical dementia. *J. Neurol.* **2013**, *260*, 1099–1103. [CrossRef] [PubMed]
15. Larner, A. History and neurological examination. In *Dementia in Clinical Practice: A Neurological Perspective*, 2nd ed.; Larner, A.J., Ed.; Springer: London, UK, 2014; pp. 41–69.
16. American Psychiatric Association. *Diagnostic and Statistical Manual of Mental Disorders*, 5th ed.; American Psychiatric Association: Arlington, VA, USA, 2013.
17. McKhann, G.M.; Knopman, D.S.; Chertkow, H.; Hyman, B.T.; Jack, C.R., Jr.; Kawas, C.H.; Klunk, W.E.; Koroshetz, W.J.; Manly, J.J.; Mayeux, R.; et al. The diagnosis of dementia due to Alzheimer's disease: Recommendations from the National Institute on Aging Alzheimer's Association workgroups on diagnostic guidelines for Alzheimer's disease. *Alzheimers Dement.* **2011**, *7*, 263–269. [CrossRef]
18. Isik, A.T.; Bozoglu, E.; Yay, A.; Soysal, P.; Ateskan, U. Which cholinesterase inhibitor is the safest for heart in elderly patients with Alzheimer's disease? *Am. J. Alzheimers Dis. Other Dement.* **2012**, *27*, 171–174. [CrossRef] [PubMed]
19. Gungen, C.; Ertan, T.; Eker, E.; Yasar, R.; Engin, F. Reliability and validity of the standardized Mini Mental State Examination in the diagnosis of mild dementia in Turkish population. *Turk. Psikiyatr. Dergisi* **2002**, *13*, 273–281.
20. Durmaz, B.; Soysal, P.; Ellidokuz, H.; Isik, A.T. Validity and reliability of geriatric depression scale-15 (short form) in Turkish older adults. *North. Clin. Istanbul* **2018**, *5*, 216–220. [CrossRef]
21. Lawton, M.P.; Brody, E.M. Assessment of older people: Selfmaintaining and instrumental activities of daily living. *Gerontologist* **1969**, *9*, 179–186. [CrossRef]
22. Mahoney, F.I.; Barthel, D. Functional evaluation: The Barthel Index: A simple index of independence useful in scoring improvement in the rehabilitation of the chronically ill. *Md. State Med. J.* **1965**, *14*, 61–65.
23. Selekler, K.; Cangöz, B.; Uluc, S. Montreal bilissel degerlendirme ölceginin hafif bilissel bozukluk ve Alzheimer hastalarini ayırtedebilme gücünün incelenmesi. *Turk. J. Geriatr.* **2010**, *13*, 166–171.
24. Kaya, D.; Isik, A.T.; Usarel, C.; Soysal, P.; Ellidokuz, H.; Grossberg, G.T. The Saint Louis University Mental Status Examination is better than the Mini-Mental State Examination to determine the cognitive impairment in Turkish elderly people. *J. Am. Med. Dir. Assoc.* **2016**, *17*, 370.e11–370.e15. [CrossRef] [PubMed]
25. Babacan-Yildiz, G.; Isik, A.T.; Ur, E.; Aydemir, E.; Ertas, C.; Cebi, M.; Soysal, P.; Gursoy, E.; Kolukisa, M.; Kocaman, G.; et al. COST: Cognitive state test, a brief screening battery for Alzheimer disease in illiterate and literate patients. *Int. Psychogeriatr.* **2013**, *25*, 403–412. [CrossRef] [PubMed]
26. Larner, A.J. Screening utility of the "attended alone" sign for subjective memory impairment. *Alzheimer Dis. Assoc. Disord.* **2014**, *28*, 364–365. [CrossRef] [PubMed]
27. Larner, A.J. 'Attended alone' sign: Validity and reliability for the exclusion of dementia. *Age Ageing* **2009**, *38*, 476–478. [CrossRef] [PubMed]
28. Bonello, M.; Larner, A.J. Applause sign: Screening utility for dementia and cognitive impairment. *Postgrad. Med.* **2016**, *128*, 250–253. [CrossRef]
29. Soysal, P.; Isik, A.T. Factors affecting sensitivity and specificity of head-turning sign in the studies. *Int. Psychogeriatr.* **2018**, *30*, 1571–1572. [CrossRef] [PubMed]
30. Takenoshita, S.; Terada, S.; Yoshida, H.; Yamaguchi, M.; Yabe, M.; Imai, N.; Horiuchi, M.; Miki, T.; Yokota, O.; Yamada, N. Validation of Addenbrooke's cognitive examination III for detecting mild cognitive impairment and dementia in Japan. *BMC Geriatr.* **2019**, *19*, 123. [CrossRef]
31. Kan, K.C.; Subramaniam, P.; Shahrizaila, N.; Kamaruzzaman, S.B.; Razali, R.; Ghazali, S.E. Validation of the Malay Version of Addenbrooke's Cognitive Examination III in Detecting Mild Cognitive Impairment and Dementia. *Dement. Geriatr. Cogn. Disord. Extra* **2019**, *9*, 66–76. [CrossRef]

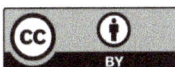

diagnostics

MDPI

Review

Test Your Memory (TYM) and Test Your Memory for Mild Cognitive Impairment (TYM-MCI): A Review and Update Including Results of Using the TYM Test in a General Neurology Clinic and Using a Telephone Version of the TYM Test

Jeremy M. Brown [1,*], Julie Wiggins [2], Kate Dawson [2], Timothy Rittman [1,2] and James B. Rowe [1,2]

[1] Department of Neurology, Box 83, Addenbrooke's Hospital, Hills Road, Cambridge CB2 2QQ, UK;
timothy.rittman@nhs.net (T.R.); james.rowe@mrc-cbu.cam.ac.uk (J.R.B.)
[2] Department of Clinical Neurosciences, University of Cambridge, Cambridge CB2 0SZ, UK;
jkw41@medschl.cam.ac.uk (J.W.); ced35@cam.ac.uk (K.D.)
* Correspondence: jmb75@medschl.cam.ac.uk

Received: 12 August 2019; Accepted: 4 September 2019; Published: 8 September 2019

Abstract: This paper summarises the current status of two novel short cognitive tests (SCT), known as Test Your Memory (TYM) and Test Your Memory for Mild Cognitive Impairment (TYM-MCI). The history of and recent research on the TYM and TYM-MCI are summarised in applications for Alzheimer's and non-Alzheimer's dementia and mild cognitive impairment. The TYM test can be used in a general neurology clinic and can help distinguish patients with Alzheimer's disease (AD) from those with no neurological cause for their memory complaints. An adapted tele-TYM test administered by telephone to patients produces scores which correlate strongly with the clinic-administered Addenbrookes Cognitive Examination revised (ACE-R) test and can identify patients with dementia. Patients with AD decline on the TYM test at a rate of 3.6–4.1 points/year.

Keywords: dementia; TYM; TYM-MCI; Alzheimer's

1. Introduction

NICE has recommended the use of the TYM test in non-specialised settings, and this paper is intended to facilitate its use and understanding [1].

1.1. The TYM Test

The original TYM test is a series of 10 cognitive tasks printed on both sides of a thin sheet of card that is filled in by a patient under minimal supervision by a non-specialist healthcare worker [2]. How much help the patient needs is used as an 11th scored "task" of the test. The TYM test can be viewed and downloaded free from the website tymtest.com. The vast majority of patients needs little help completing the TYM test and this allows the supervising health worker to continue to perform other tasks at the same time, e.g., welcoming patients to the clinic, booking patients in and out, or filling in a scan form. Scoring the TYM test takes approximately two minutes. The TYM test therefore takes a minimal amount of medical time to administer. Much of the administration and scoring of the test is intuitive, meaning staff need minimal training to supervise and score the test. JMB (Jeremy M. Brown) has successfully taught many nurses at the Queen Elizabeth Hospital, King's Lynn, and elsewhere to supervise the test at the start of the clinic, even if they have no experience of memory clinics. It is possible to obtain valid results with patients' relatives rather than health professionals supervising the test [3]. A sheet is available from the website tymtest.com to aid scoring and more detailed scoring sheets are available from JMB.

The 11 tasks cover a wide range of cognitive skills similar to those tested by the Addenbrookes Cognitive Examinations (ACE) [4–6] and in all our studies the TYM score is very strongly correlated to the ACE-R (Addenbrookes Cognitive Examination Revised) score (with high Pearson co-efficient). The ACE-R and ACE-III are the gold standard short cognitive tests in use in memory clinics, and are widely used throughout the world. The TYM test is scored out of 50 and the ACE-R and ACE-III are scored out of 100; doubling the TYM score will give a good estimate of the ACE-R or ACE-III score.

1.2. Domains of the TYM Test

1. Orientation to time and person (orientation)—scored out of 10
2. Copying a sentence (copying)—scored out of 2
3. Recall of facts (facts)—scored out of 3
4. Arithmetic (sums)—scored out of 4
5. Animal Fluencies (fluencies)—scored out of 4
6. Similarities—scored out of 4
7. Naming—scored out of 5
8. Spotting the letter W (visuospatial 1)—scored out of 3
9. Completing a clock (visuospatial 2)—scored out of 4
10. Recall of the sentence (recall)—scored out of 6
11. Help needed to complete the test (help)—scored out of 5

2. History

The TYM test was invented and developed by the author from 2007 to 2009 and the original validation paper was published in the BMJ (British Medical Journal) in 2009 [2]. This showed that the TYM test detected the majority of patients with Alzheimer's disease. There was considerable initial publicity and interest and almost immediately a large number of validation projects began throughout the world. Many of these have now been published in peer-reviewed journals. A table giving a review of these papers was included in a chapter in 2015, and since then more validation studies have been published. Table 1 includes a summary of the results of all of these studies, which include over 4000 individuals. The protocols for the different studies vary and the populations studied were very different, so there is limited value in comparing sensitivities and specificities.

All of the studies published are positive, demonstrating that the TYM test is a good short cognitive test for the detection of dementia in a wide range of cultures, in different languages, and using different alphabets. The test was developed in the United Kingdom and does show a cultural bias. This has necessitated some country-specific modifications of the TYM test, which are usually minor, e.g., changing important national dates or the letter for animal fluencies. The sentence about "stout shoes" is very British and the alternative sentence "Great cooks always bake chocolate cakes" has been used in several validations. It is important that the sentence is not a well-known phrase and it needs to be counter-intuitive to avoid a patient guessing the end by remembering the first couple of words. The sentence should not be directly translated, as to do so may undermine its critical features for cognitive assessment. Information on how to adapt the TYM test for different languages is available from JMB.

The tymtest.com website was launched in 2010. Health professionals can view the test and download the TYM test from the site free of charge for healthcare and research purposes. They can also download scoring instructions and advice on how to administer the test. The website continues to be widely used and the TYM test has now been downloaded more than 20,500 times from the website.

The website is currently being upgraded and videos will be added to aid the use and standardisation of the TYM test. The TYM-MCI will also be available from the site.

Table 1. Summary of TYM validation studies.

Country	First Author Reference	Numbers Recruited	Setting and Disease	Cut off Used Sensitivity/Specificity or Other Parameter
Japan	Hanyui [7]	159	Memory Clinic AD	Cut off varied Sensitivity 0.96 Specificity 0.88
Japan	Kotuku [8]	334	Memory Clinic AD	Cut off 42 Sensitivity 0.82 Specificity 0.72
United Kingdom	Hancock [3]	224	2 Memory Clinics Dementia	Cut off 30 Sensitivity 0.73 Specificity 0.88
Poland	Szczesniak [9]	225	Memory Clinic AD	Cut off 39 Sensitivity 0.91 Specificity 0.90
Poland	Derkacz [10]	65	Memory Clinic	Cut off 36 Improvement on MMSE (mini-mental state examination)
France	Postel-Vinay [11]	201	Memory Clinic Dementia	Cut off 39 Sensitivity 0.90 Specificity
Greece	Iatraki [12,13]	373	Community and Neurology Clinic Dementia	Cut off varied Sensitivity 0.82 (0.80) Specificity 0.71 (0.77)
South Africa	Van Schalkwyk [14]	100	Primary Care Dementia	Strong correlation with MMSE
Chile Spanish	Munoz-Neira [15]	74	Memory Clinic Dementia	Cut off 39 Specificity 0.93 Sensitivity 0.82
Netherlands	Koekkoek [16]	86	Memory Clinic	AUC = 0.88 Correlated with neuropsychological tests
Netherlands	Van der Zande [17]		Memory Clinic Dementia	Better than MMSE
Turkey	Mavis [18]	395	Memory Clinic Dementia	Cut off 34 Sensitivity 0.97 Specificity 0.96
Argentina Spanish	Serrani [19]	300	Memory Clinic Dementia	Cut off 40 Sensitivity 0.84 Specificity 0.95
Norway	Breitve [20]	33	Memory Clinic	Cut off 42 Specificity 0.84 Sensitivity 1.00 For dementia
Spain	Ferrero-Arias [21]	1049	Neurology Clinic Dementia	Cut off 36 Sensitivity 0.94 Specificity 0.89 For dementia
Iran	Salami [22]	175	Community AD	Cut off 31 Sensitivity 0.9 Specificity 1.0
EgyptArabic	Abd-Al-Atty [23]	206	Hospital Dementia	Cut off 39/40 in well-educated patients only. Sensitivity 0.80 Specificity 0.97
China Mandarin	Xuemei [24]	237	Neurology Clinic AD	Cut off 39.5 Sensitivity 0.95 Specificity 0.95
Hungary	Kolozsvari [25]	50	Community AD	Cut off 35/36 Sensitivity 0.94 Specificity 0.94
Singapore	Dong [26]	90	Memory Clinic AD	Cut off 38 As good as MOCA (Montreal Cognitive Assessment) Better than MMSE AUC 0.96

2.1. TYM Tests for Non-Alzheimer's Dementia

Further studies on the TYM test by the author have also confirmed the initial findings [27]. Recently the author published a validation study of the TYM test in non-Alzheimer's dementia [28]. These included the behavioural variant of frontotemporal dementia, semantic dementia, vascular dementia, progressive non-fluent aphasia, corticobasal syndrome, progressive supranuclear palsy and atypical focal presentations of Alzheimer's disease (posterior cortical atrophy and logopaenic aphasia).

The TYM test was a useful test in detecting each of these different dementia types. The standard TYM test (cut off 42) detected 80% of non-Alzheimer's or atypical Alzheimer's dementia, whereas the ACE-R (cut off 82) detected 69% of cases and the MMSE (Mini-mental state examination) (cut off 23) detected only 27%. When grouping all of the different diseases together, the TYM test had a positive predictive value of 0.80 and a negative predictive value of 0.84, with an area under the ROC curve of 0.89, similar to its accuracy at detection of typical Alzheimer's disease. The pattern of scoring on the TYM test differed between conditions, and the pattern of deficits can be useful in supporting a clinical diagnosis, particularly for semantic dementia and posterior cortical atrophy.

2.2. The TYM-MCI

The TYM test has been shown to be useful in the detection of both Alzheimer's and non-Alzheimer's dementia. Empirically it is unlikely to be as useful in detecting amnestic mild cognitive impairment, an important role in the memory clinic, as it has 9 points for memory, and so a patient with single cognitive domain deficits in memory may need to score just 2/9 in order for them to reach the threshold of 43/50.

The detection of early or mild clinical cases of aMCI (amnestic Mild Cognitive Impairment) or early symptomatic AD is important, particularly as disease modifying treatments are developed. JMB recognised the need for a short cognitive test aimed at better sensitivity to aMCI and this led to the TYM-MCI test. During its development, the TYM-MCI was known first as the Hard TYM (H-TYM) or the Tricky TYM. The current and more formal name TYM-MCI is the most apt name, describing exactly what it does—it detects mild cognitive impairment.

The TYM-MCI is the first short cognitive test to examine both visual and verbal episodic memory. It looks rather similar to the TYM test and will be available shortly on the website tymtest.com. However, the usage of the TYM-MCI is very different from the TYM test—the TYM-MCI is administered by a health professional. The administration takes approximately 7 minutes. The TYM-MCI should only be used for the detection of aMCI or mild AD (unlike the TYM test, which can be used in many clinical scenarios), and the patient should have completed and performed well on a standard SCT (either TYM or other appropriate SCT) prior to attempting the TYM-MCI. It can be run immediately following the standard TYM in a clinic setting. As the diagnostic value rests on the patient's recall of recently learnt visual and verbal information, only the recall tasks on page 2 are scored. The scoring system will be released shortly on the website tymtest.com and is available from JMB. Visual recall and verbal recall are both scored out of 15, giving a maximum total score of 30.

Two validation studies of the TYM-MCI have been reported [29,30] and both showed very striking results. The initial validation compared the TYM-MCI scores in patients with mild AD and normal controls [29]. This kind of validation study, a proof of principle, sets a fairly low bar, which the TYM-MCI nonetheless passed very easily and with very clear results. Patients with mild AD scored 6.7/30 on the TYM-MCI compared to normal controls who scored 20.4/30. The area under the ROC (receiver operating characteristic) curve was 0.99. The results were particularly impressive for recall of visual encoded information with both a modal and median score of 0/15 for patients with mild AD or aMCI compared to a mean of 10/15 for the controls. The greater deficit in visual recall may reflect preferential involvement of recall of visual information in the earliest stages of AD or may reflect that it is a more difficult sub-test of the TYM-MCI than the recall of verbally encoded information. One other H-TYM study confirmed it was a useful test [31].

The second validation study [30] was more clinically relevant, examining the usefulness of the TYM-MCI in the separation of patients with aMCI or mild AD from patients presenting to the same memory clinic with memory complaints that were felt not to have a neurological cause (subjective memory complaints). These patients could be "worried well", depressed, or have conditions such as obstructive sleep apnoea. The study was a thorough assessment of the TYM-MCI, for example including only patients who scored in the normal range on the MMSE.

The TYM-MCI performed very well, with a specificity of 0.79 and a sensitivity of 0.91 in distinguishing the two groups of patients. An important result of this study was that the TYM-MCI was shown to provide additional information to the ACE-R and add information to the overall clinical assessment. Three useful practical conclusions from this paper were:

1. The combination of the TYM-MCI with the ACE-R detects virtually all cases of aMCI or mild AD.

2.   The TYM-MCI is a useful test in patients with borderline ACE-R scores. A total of 72% of patients with aMCI or mild AD who had a borderline score on the ACE-R (scoring between the 2 thresholds of 82 and 89) were detected on the TYM-MCI and 79% of patients with subjective memory complaints and a borderline ACE-R score passed the TYM-MCI.

3.   Patients initially felt to have subjective memory problems who were later re-diagnosed with organic aMCI scored poorly on their initial TYM-MCI (mean score 9.8/30).

The TYM-MCI is now used routinely in the Addenbrooke's memory clinic for patients whom we suspect have early AD/aMCI as the cause of their memory problems but whom have scored well (>82/100) on the ACE-R.

2.3. TYM Testing in a Non-Specialised Clinical Settings

The TYM was designed for use in non-specialised clinics and NICE (National Institute for Health and Care Excellence) has recommended the use of the TYM test in non-specialised settings [1]. The validation research studies were undertaken in primary, secondary, and tertiary care settings. In this section, we outline the use of TYM testing in a NHS (National Health Service) Trust hospital's general neurology clinic at Queen Elizabeth Hospital, King's Lynn, United Kingdom.

Research validation of the TYM test in general clinics has different endpoints to the memory clinical validation against ACE-R or ACE-III and multidisciplinary team review. In the generalist setting, there is often no definitive "memory" outcome to the consultation. However, feedback on its widespread use suggests that it does provide useful information. One study has reported on the results of TYM testing in a general neurology clinic [21], but again outcomes regarding diagnostic accuracy are difficult to assess. Here we describe our own work on the TYM test in general neurology clinics.

Materials and Methods: Between January 2013 and August 2018, a total of 938 TYM tests were administered in general neurology clinics at Queen Elizabeth Hospital, King's Lynn, United Kingdom. The age of the patients tested ranged from 18 to 93 years of age. The average age was 65.9 years. The majority of TYM tests were performed on patients with memory complaints either as a sole problem or as part of a neurological illness, such as Parkinson's disease, multiple sclerosis or epilepsy. The general clinic nurses supervised the TYM tests with minimal training and in addition to their usual clinic duties. There were no major problems or complaints from supervising staff or patients.

Results: Many of the diagnoses recorded in the letters were not definitive and patients were not necessarily followed-up, so we do not present its diagnostic accuracy against a gold standard of specialist review and extensive investigations. The final diagnosis could not be determined for many patients and these individuals are not included in the analysis. These data are therefore "pragmatic" and embedded in a real-world setting. The diagnoses were clinical and not made according to international criteria, so detailed analysis is not appropriate. The data are summarized in Table 2.

Table 2. Characteristics and TYM test results of patients with various diseases in a general neurology clinic. The diagnoses were clinical.

Diagnosis	No.	Age Range Years	Age: Mean and SD Years	TYM Score Range	TYM: Mean and SD
Clinical Alzheimer's disease	81	48–89	74.7 ± 9.1	0–48	29.6 ± 11.1
Clinical Parkinson's disease	132	46–90	71.2 ± 9.9	21–50	40.2 ± 7.3
Clinical dementia with Lewy bodies	31	68–84	75.9 ± 5.0	20–46	35.2 ± 7.6
Clinical MCI (Mild Cognitive Impairment)	43	52–86	71.7 ± 9.5	24–49	40.2 ± 7.7
Clinical Epilepsy	30	21–73	58.0 ± 18.1	26–49	39.7 ± 7.2
Subjective memory loss	116	23–88	57.6 ± 14.3	24–50	42.3 ± 5.3

Patients with a clinical diagnosis of Alzheimer's disease had significantly lower TYM scores than those with subjective memory loss ($p < 0.001$)

2.4. Rates of Change in Clinical Alzheimer's Disease, Clinical Parkinson's Disease and Patients Felt to Have Subjective Memory Complaints

Seventeen patients with a final diagnosis of clinical Alzheimer's disease completed the TYM test on more than one visit (follow-up 6–50 months). The rate of decline was variable between individuals and there was no clear relationship to disease severity. The mean rate of deterioration was 4.1 points/year, in keeping with a typical rate of decline of 10 points per year on the ACE-R.

Twenty patients with clinical Parkinson's disease had TYM tests on more than one visit (range 5–60 months). Four patients had an improvement in their score, 4 scored the same, and 12/20 (60%) showed a decline. The rate of decline was variable between individuals and there was no clear relationship to disease severity. Overall, the rate of decline in TYM scores in PD was 1.4 points/year.

Twenty-five patients with a final baseline diagnosis of subjective memory problems completed the TYM test on more than one visit (follow-up 4–50 months). Interestingly, 18/25 showed a small improvement in their TYM score, 4 had the same score, and only 3 declined. The mean rate of change in the TYM score was plus 1.2 points/year. It seems most likely that a mild practice effect was responsible for the improvement in TYM scores.

3. Conclusions

The TYM test has been used since 2013 without any complications or complaints. Patients were tested because they had memory complaints or were suspected of having cognitive problems. The major categories of patients were those suspected of having Alzheimer's disease or other dementia, patients with subjective memory problems, Parkinson's disease, epilepsy and mild cognitive impairment. In patients who were followed-up with, the TYM test proved very useful, as patients with AD declined at an average rate of 4.1 points per year, whereas patients with subjective complaints tended to show a small increase in TYM scores with time. Patients with Parkinson's disease had an average score of 40.2/50 on the TYM test—below the threshold for supporting a diagnosis of dementia. PD patients did decline on the TYM test but at a much slower rate than patients with AD (1.4 points/year). The TYM test reveals memory problems in the other groups of patients seen in a General Neurology clinic but the numbers of these patients were too small to make clear conclusions.

3.1. The Telephone TYM or Tele-TYM

While supervised TYM testing in a clinic setting works well, there are situations where a remote assessment would be helpful, such as pre-admission clerking or follow-up. Patients may also be more relaxed and perform better at home, while it could save an outpatient appointment or allow better planning of appointments (e.g., to decide who might benefit from a pre-clinic brain scan). In principle, one could assess cognitive function over the telephone or using an internet-based consultation. Cognitive testing of patients by telephone is not straightforward but could bring advantages to both health care professionals and patients. A telephone TYM test could be used to help assess the response of a patient to a cholinesterase inhibitor and save a journey to outpatients.

As the TYM test is filled in by the patient, it has the potential to be administered by telephone, and we investigated this in a pilot study in 2017.

The protocol was as follows. Patients who were due to be seen in a specialised memory clinic in approximately 6 weeks were contacted by a research nurse and offered the chance to participate in the telephone TYM study. If they consented to the trial, a date about 2 weeks in advance of the clinic was agreed. They were asked to ensure that a relative or friend who was able to help them was available at that time.

They were sent an envelope with details of the trial, including an envelope containing the TYM test, which was marked "not to be opened before nurse phones". There was also a stamped, addressed envelope for the patient to return the completed test to the clinic nurse.

The nurse would phone the patient at the agreed time. She would ask them to sit down in a comfortable chair at a table with their reading glasses, a pen and a helper. They were then asked to open the envelope. The nurse encouraged them to fill in the TYM test themselves as much as possible but remained on the end of the phone and provided assistance or reassurance when required. She recorded how much time and help the patient needed. She reminded them to remember the sentence at the end of page 1 and not to turn the page back. Once they finished, the nurse asked them to place the completed TYM test in the envelope and post it to her.

When the patient came to the clinic they had the usual assessment, which includes seeing an experienced nurse who would administer the ACE-R and MMSE, followed by a neurologist, imaging as required, and multidisciplinary team review. Results of the telephone TYM test were then compared to the ACE-R and MMSE results. A subset of the patients had an additional TYM test in the clinic (often a different version of the TYM test, such as the TYM-B (Test Your Memory version B). Practice effects can be seen in the TYM test if it is administered twice at short intervals. This can be only partially alleviated by using a different version of the TYM test and we normally do not repeat the TYM test at an interval of less than 3 months.

117 patients were recruited. Of these, 16 failed to complete the TYM test or did not attend their clinic appointment. Additionally, 22 patients had diagnoses such as Parkinson's disease, stroke or epilepsy which may or may not be associated with an organic dementia, and so were not included in the analysis. A total of 81 patients were included in the analysis—43 patients were felt to have subjective memory problems with no identified neurological cause for their memory problems after their assessment by a consultant with a special interest in cognition; 38 patients were given organic cognitive diagnoses. The breakdown of the organic cases was: mild cognitive impairment, 18; Alzheimer's disease, 9; unspecified organic dementia, 5; semantic dementia, 2; mixed dementia, 2; dementia with Lewy bodies, 1; progressive supranuclear palsy, 1.

Patients with an organic cause for their memory problems were significantly older than patients with subjective memory complaints. However, in this study there was no correlation between TYM score and age. Patients with organic disease scored lower in all three cognitive tests than those with subjective memory complaints but no underlying neurological disease (Table 3). There was a strong correlation between the telephone TYM score and the clinic ACE-R score in both groups (Pearson $r = 0.83$ organic, $r = 0.60$ subjective memory complaints). There were no complications from the study and no complaints from the patients concerning the telephone testing. Very occasionally the nurse suspected some cheating.

Table 3. Telephone TYM scores, clinic ACE-R (Addenbrooke's Cognitive Examination Revised) and clinic MMSE scores in patients with organic dementia or MCI and no organic dementia.

Characteristics	Organic Dementia/MCI	Subjective Memory Complaints
Number in study	38	43
Mean age	69.7	60.5
Telephone TYM score	36.9	43.8
Clinic ACE-R score	71.4	87.6
Clinic MMSE	24.5	27.7

This study shows that it is possible to administer the TYM test over the telephone. The telephone TYM test shows very good correlation with an ACE-R test administered by an experienced ACE tester in clinic. Used alone as a cognitive test the tele-TYM shows a sensitivity of 78% and specificity of 69%, with a cut-off set at ≥43. Comparing the patients with organic and subjective memory diagnoses, the tele-TYM score was significantly lower in the organic group ($p < 0.001$, Wilcoxon rank sum test, corrected for multiple comparisons). The results are summarised in Table 4 below.

Table 4. Results of the Telephone TYM study.

Score	Organics Mean	Subjective Memory Complaints Mean	*p* Value Corrected
Tele-TYM overall score	36.9	43.8	<0.001
Orientation	8.9	9.7	0.011
Copy	1.5	1.8	ns
Facts	1.5	2.2	ns
Sums	3.3	3.6	ns
Fluencies	2.2	3.2	0.008
Similarities	3.1	3.5	ns
Naming	4.5	4.6	ns
Visuospatial 1	1.8	2.4	ns
Visuospatial 2	2.9	3.7	0.006
Recall	2.4	4.0	ns
Help	4.7	5.0	0.01

Note: ns = non-significant.

3.2. Longitudinal TYM Studies

Thirty-four patients with Alzheimer's disease had more than 1 TYM test administered in the Cambridge memory clinic with an interval of between 2 months and 52 months (mean 15 months). There was an average decline in the TYM test of 3.6 points per year.

3.3. TYM Passers with a Diagnosis of Amnestic Mild Cognitive Impairment

One of the drawbacks of the TYM test is that it does not reliably detect patients with amnestic mild cognitive impairment or very mild Alzheimer's disease on total score. To examine this further we selected the 46 patients with a diagnosis of aMCI or mild AD who passed the TYM test and compared them to 157 normal controls. Their results are shown in Table 5.

Table 5. Comparison of TYM and TYM subtest scores in patients with aMCI (amnestic mild cognitive impairment) who passed the TYM test compared to controls.

Characteristic	aMCI	Percentage	Controls	Percentage	*p* = corrected
n =	46		157		
Age	68.3		67.5		ns
TYM total/50	45.0	90	46	92	ns
Orientation/10	9.9	99	9.8	98	ns
Copying/2	2.0	98	1.8	90	ns
Facts/3	2.4	81	2.6	87	ns
Sums/4	3.2	81	3.7	93	ns
Fluencies/4	3.4	84	3.4	85	ns
Similarities/4	3.8	94	3.3	83	ns
Naming/5	4.9	99	4.9	98	ns
Visuospatial 1/3	2.8	92	2.8	92	ns
Visuospatial 2/4	3.1	78	3.7	93	ns
Recall/6	3.5	58	5.0	83	<0.001
Help/5	4.7	95	5.0	100	<0.001

4. Discussion

We looked retrospectively to see whether the pattern of TYM scoring can help distinguish patients with mild amnestic AD who pass the TYM test from controls. The only significant differences between the 2 groups were in recall and help given. Patients with aMCI tended to score comparatively poorly on the second page of the TYM test. One other study [32] has examined the value of the TYM test in the diagnosis of aMCI in a community-based cohort of patients and showed that the TYM test had a specificity of 0.87 and sensitivity of 0.63 in the diagnosis of aMCI.

5. Conclusions

1.   The TYM test is a useful short cognitive test in the support of a diagnosis of AD.
2.   The TYM test detects a majority of patients with non-Alzheimer's dementia and unusual presentations of AD.
3.   The usefulness of the TYM test has been shown in over 20 published studies in peer-reviewed journals covering different languages, cultures and alphabets.
4.   Patients with AD show a decline on the TYM test of 3.6 and 4.1 points/year in two different studies.
5.   The TYM test can be used in a general neurology clinic. Patients with AD score significantly lower on the TYM test than patients with no identified neurological cause for their subjective memory problems. Follow-up TYM testing shows that patients with AD decline at an average rate of 4.1 points per year, whilst the patients with subjective memory complaints show a small improvement on average.
6.   The TYM test can be used over the telephone with results that correlate with clinic-administered tests, and show a significant difference between patients with organic disease and those with no neurological cause for their subjective memory problems.
7.   Patients with amnestic MCI score more poorly than controls on recall and help given on subtests of the TYM.
8.   The TYM-MCI is a short cognitive test that can support a clinical diagnosis of mild AD and amnestic MCI.

JMB can be contacted via the website tymtest.com.

Author Contributions: Formal analysis, T.R.; investigation, J.M.B., J.W., and K.D.; project administration, J.B.R.; writing—original draft, J.M.B.

Funding: This work was co-funded by the NIHR Cambridge Biomedical Research Centre and the Wellcome Trust (JBR:103838).

Conflicts of Interest: The authors declare no conflict of interest.

References

1.   National Institute for Health and Care Excellence, London. *Dementia: Assessment, Management and Support for People Living with Dementia and Their Carers*; National Institute for Health and Care Excellence (UK): London, UK, 2018.
2.   Brown, J.M.; Pengas, G.; Dawson, K.; Brown, L.A.; Clatworthy, P. Self-administered cognitive screening test (TYM) for detection of Alzheimer's disease: Cross sectional study. *BMJ* **2009**, *338*, b2030. [CrossRef]
3.   Hancock, P.; Larner, A.J. Test Your Memory: Diagnostic utility in a memory clinic population. *Int. J. Geriatr. Psychiatry* **2011**, *26*, 976–980. [CrossRef] [PubMed]
4.   Mathuranath, P.S.; Nestor, P.J.; Berrios, G.E.; Rakowicz, W.; Hodges, J. A brief cognitive test battery to differentiate Alzheimer's disease and frontotemporal dementia. *Neurology* **2000**, *55*, 1613–1620. [CrossRef] [PubMed]
5.   Mioshi, E.; Dawson, K.; Mitchell, J.; Arnold, R.; Hodges, J. The Addenbrooke's cognitive examination revised (ACE-R). A brief cognitive test battery for dementia screening. *Int. J. Geriatr. Psychiatry* **2006**, *21*, 1078–1085. [CrossRef] [PubMed]
6.   Hodges, J.R.; Larner, A.J. Addenbrooke's Cognitive Examinations: ACE, ACE-R, ACE-111, ACE app and M-ACE. In *Cognitive Screening Instruments a Practical Approach.*, 2nd ed.; Larner, A.J., Ed.; Springer: London, UK, 2017; pp. 109–137.
7.   Hanyu, H.; Maezone, M.; Sakurai, H.; Kume, K.; Kanetaka, H.; Iwamoto, T. Japanese version of the Test Your Memory as a screening test in a Japanese memory clinic. *Psychiatry Res.* **2011**, *190*, 145–148. [CrossRef] [PubMed]
8.   Kutoku, Y.; Oshsawa, Y.; Kushida, R.; Fuki, Y.; Izawa, N.; Rikimaru, M.; Miyazaki, Y.; Kurokawa, K.; Murakami, T.; Sunada, Y. Diagnostic utility of the Japanese version of Test Your Memory (TYM-J) for Alzheimer's disease. *Kawasaki Med. J.* **2011**, *37*, 177–184.

9. Szczesniak, D.; Wojtynska, R.; Rymaszewska, J. Test Your Memory (TYM) as a screening instrument in clinical practice—the Polish validation study. *Aging Ment. Health* **2013**, *17*, 863–868. [CrossRef]

10. Derkacz, M.; Chmiel-Perzynska, I.; Kowal, A.; Pawlos, J.; Michalojic-Derkacz, M.; Olajossy, M.; Marczewski, K. Tym Test—Novel diagnostic tool to assess cognitive functions—study on inhabitants of social welfare house. *Curr. Probl. Psychiatry* **2011**, *12*, 152–159.

11. Postel-Vinay, N.; Hanon, O.; Clerson, P.; Brown, J.; Menard, J.; Paillaud, E.; Alonso, E.; Pasquier, F.; Pariel, S.; Belliard, S.; et al. Validation of the Test Your Memory (F-TYM Test) in a French memory clinic population. *Clin. Neuropsychol.* **2014**, *28*, 994–1007. [CrossRef]

12. Iatraki, E.; Simos, P.; Lionis, C.; Zaganas, I.; Symvoulakis, E.; Papastefanakis, E.; Panagiotakis, S.; Pantelidakis, H.; Papadopoulos, K.; Tziraki, C. Cultural adaption, standardization and clinical validity of the Test Your Memory dementia screening instrument in Greek. *Dement. Geriatr. Cogn. Disord.* **2014**, *37*, 163–180. [CrossRef]

13. Iatraki, E.; Simos, P.; Bertias, A.; Duijker, G.; Zagamas, I.; Tziraki, C.; Vgontzas, A.; Lionis, C.; Thalis Primary Health Care Research Team/Network. Cognitive screening tools for primary care settings: Examining the "Test Your Memory" and "General Practice Assessment of Cognition" tools in a rural aging population in Greece. *Eur. J. Gen. Pract.* **2017**, *23*, 172–179. [CrossRef] [PubMed]

14. Van Schalkwyk, G.; Botha, H.; Seedat, S. Comparison of 2 dementia screeners, the Test Your Memory Test and the Mini-Mental State Examination, in a Primary Care Setting. *J. Geriatr. Psychiatry Neurol.* **2012**, *25*, 85–88. [CrossRef] [PubMed]

15. Munoz-Neira, C.; Chaparro, F.; Delgado, C.; Brown, J.; Slachevsky, A. Test Your Memory—Spanish version (TYM-S): A validation study of a self-administered cognitive screening test. *Int. J. Geriatr. Psychiatry* **2014**, *29*, 730–740. [CrossRef] [PubMed]

16. Koekkoek, P.; Rutten, G.; van der Berg, E.; van Sonsbeek, S.; Gorter, K.; Kappelle, L.; Biessels, G. The "Test Your Memory" test performs better than the MMSE in a population without known cognitive dysfunction. *J. Neurol. Sci.* **2013**, *328*, 92–97. [CrossRef] [PubMed]

17. Van de Zande, E.; Van de Nes, J.; Jansen, I.; van den Berg, M.; Zwart, A.; Bimmel, D.; Rijkers, G.; Andringa, G. The Test Your Memory (TYM) Test Outperforms the MMSE in the Detection of MCI and Dementia. *Curr. Alz. Res.* **2017**, *14*, 598–607. [CrossRef] [PubMed]

18. Mavis, I.; Ozbabalik Adapinar, B.; Yenilmez, C.; Aydin, A.; OLgun, E.; Bal, C. Test your memory—Turkish version. *Turk. J. Med. Sci.* **2015**, *45*, 1178–1185. [PubMed]

19. Serrani, D. Spanish validation of the TYM Test for dementia screening in the Argentine population. *Univ. Psychol.* **2014**, *13*, 265–284.

20. Breitve, M.; Chwiszuk, L.; Hynninen, M. A Norwegian pilot study of the TYM test. An alternative to the Norwegian MMSE. *Tidsskr. Nor. Psykologforening* **2015**, *52*, 49–53.

21. Ferrero-Arias, J.; Turrion-Rojo, M. Validation of a Spanish version of the Test Your Memory. *Neurologia* **2016**, *31*, 33–42. [CrossRef]

22. Salami, M.; Alinaghipour, A.; Daneshvar, R.; Hamidi, G.; Agahi, A.; Soheili, M.; Akbari, H.; Taba, S. Adapted MMSE and TYM cognitive tests: How much powerful in screening for Alzheimer's disease in Iranian people. *Aging Ment. Health* **2019**. [CrossRef]

23. Abd-Al-Atty, M.; Abou-Hashem, R.; Abd El Gawad, W.; Elgazzar, Y. Test Your Memory, Arabic Version. Is it practical in a different culture? *J. Am. Geriatr. Soc.* **2012**, *60*, 596–597. [CrossRef] [PubMed]

24. Xuemei, L.; Zhang, J.; Zhu, J.; Zhang, Y.; Zhang, W.; Tin, D. Construct validity and reliability of the Test Your Memory Chinese version in older neurology outpatient attendees. *Int. J. Ment. Health Sys.* **2018**, *12*, 64.

25. Kolozsvari, L.; Kovacs, Z.; Szollosi, G.; Frecska, E.; Egerhazi, A. Validation of the Hungarian version of the Test Your Memory. *Ideggyogy* **2017**, *70*, 267–272. [CrossRef]

26. Dong, Y.; Ling, T.; Ng, K.; Wang, A.; Wan, E.; Merchant, R.; Venketasubramanian, N.; Chen, C.; Amahendran, R.; Collinson, S. The Clinical Utility of the TYM and RBANS in a One-Stop Memory Clinic in Singapore: A Pilot Study. *J. Geriatr. Psychiatry Neurol.* **2019**, *32*, 68–73. [CrossRef] [PubMed]

27. Brown, J.M. TYM (Test Your Memory) Testing. In *Cognitive Screening Instruments. A Practical Approach*, 2nd ed.; Larner, A.J., Ed.; Springer: London, UK, 2017; pp. 209–229.

28. Brown, J.; Wiggins, J.; Lansdall, C.J.; Dawson, K.; Rittman, T.; Rowe, J. Test Your Memory: Diagnostic evaluation of patients with non-Alzheimer dementias. *J. Neurol.* **2019**. [CrossRef] [PubMed]

29. Brown, J.; Wiggins, J.; Dong, H.; Harvey, R.; Richardson, F.; Hunter, K.; Dawson, K.; Parker, R. The hard Test Your Memory. Evaluation of a short cognitive test to detect mild Alzheimer's disease and amnestic mild cognitive impairment. *Int. J. Geriatr. Psychaitry* **2014**, *29*, 272–280. [CrossRef]

30. Brown, J.; Lansdall, C.J.; Wiggins, J.; Dawson, K.; Hunter, K.; Rowe, J.; Parker, R. The Test Your Memory for Mild Cognitive Impairment (TYM-MCI). *J. Neurol. Neurosurg. Psychiatry* **2017**, *88*, 1045–1051. [CrossRef]

31. Larner, A.J. Hard TYM: A pragmatic study. *Int. J. Geriatr. Psychiatry* **2015**, *30*, 330–331. [CrossRef]

32. Ozer, S.; Noonan, K.; Burke, M.; Young, J.; Barber, S.; Forster, A.; Jones, R. The validity of the Memory Alteration Test and the Test Your Memory test for community-based identification of amnestic mild cognitive impairment. *Alzheimers Dement.* **2016**, *12*, 987–995. [CrossRef]

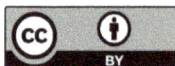

Article

Codex (Cognitive Disorders Examination) Decision Tree Modified for the Detection of Dementia and MCI

Besa Ziso and Andrew J. Larner *

Cognitive Function Clinic, Walton Centre for Neurology and Neurosurgery, Liverpool L9 7LJ, UK;
besa.Ziso@thewaltoncentre.nhs.uk
* Correspondence: A.J.Larner@thewaltoncentre.nhs.uk

Received: 26 March 2019; Accepted: 30 May 2019; Published: 1 June 2019

Abstract: Many cognitive screening instruments are available to assess patients with cognitive symptoms in whom a diagnosis of dementia or mild cognitive impairment is being considered. Most are quantitative scales with specified cut-off values. In contrast, the cognitive disorders examination or Codex is a two-step decision tree which incorporates components from the Mini-Mental State Examination (MMSE) (three word recall, spatial orientation) along with a simplified clock drawing test to produce categorical outcomes defining the probability of dementia diagnosis and, by implication, directing clinician response (reassurance, monitoring, further investigation, immediate treatment). Codex has been shown to have high sensitivity and specificity for dementia diagnosis but is less sensitive for the diagnosis of mild cognitive impairment (MCI). We examined minor modifications to the Codex decision tree to try to improve its sensitivity for the diagnosis of MCI, based on data extracted from studies of two other cognitive screening instruments, the Montreal Cognitive Assessment and Free-Cog, which are more stringent than MMSE in their tests of delayed recall. Neither modification proved of diagnostic value for mild cognitive impairment. Possible explanations for this failure are considered.

Keywords: Codex; decision tree; dementia; Free-Cog; MoCA; mild cognitive impairment; sensitivity and specificity

---

1. Introduction

The cognitive disorders examination or Codex for the detection of dementia described by Belmin et al. [1,2] is a two-step decision tree for diagnostic prediction, developed by identifying independent variables related to dementia using a multivariable logistic model. Binary recursive partitioning incorporated the three-word recall and spatial orientation components from the Mini-Mental State Examination (MMSE) [3] along with a simplified clock drawing test (sCDT, scored 1 or 0, respectively, normal and abnormal) to produce four terminal nodes, the endpoint values having different probabilities of dementia diagnosis (categories A–D, respectively, with very low, low, high, and very high probability of dementia; Figure 1a). Codex takes around three minutes to perform. In the index study, Codex had both high sensitivity and specificity for the diagnosis of dementia (0.92 and 0.85, respectively) [1].

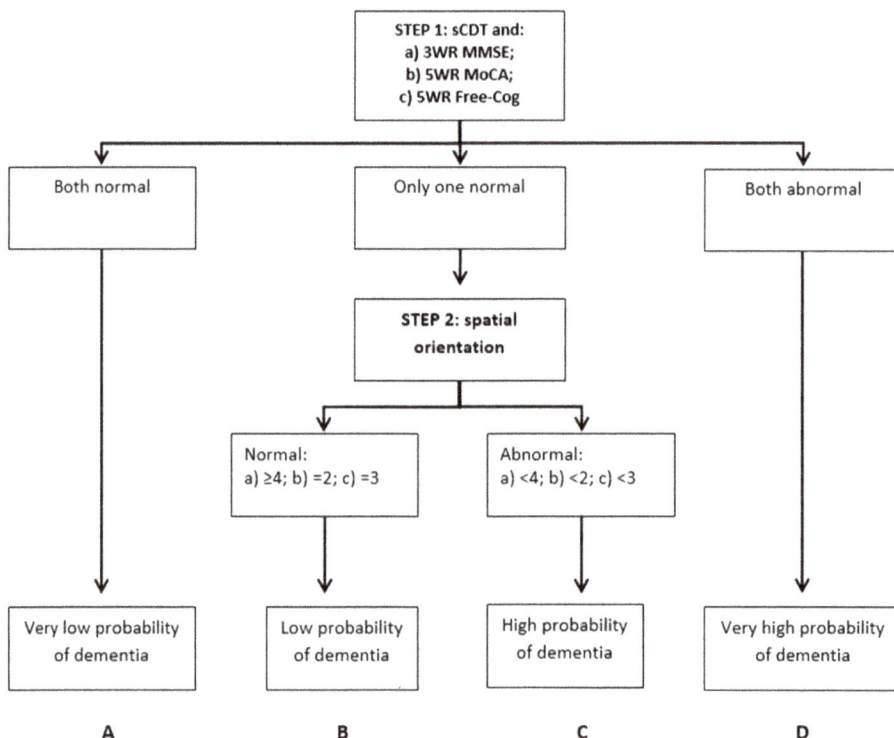

Figure 1. Codex decision tree: (**a**) Original Codex categories (from Belmin et al. 2007 [1]); (**b**) modified Codex categories from MoCA; (**c**) modified Codex categories from Free-Cog.

An independent pragmatic test accuracy study of Codex, undertaken by Ziso and Larner in a dedicated cognitive disorders clinic in a secondary care setting [4–6], confirmed good sensitivity and specificity for dementia diagnosis (0.84 and 0.82, respectively), as did a proof of concept study of a Greek translation of Codex based in a primary care setting (sensitivity 0.94, specificity 0.89) [7].

Codex has also found other applications, for example, in predicting postoperative delirium in patients undergoing femoral fracture repair [8] and in monitoring cognitive impairment before and after cochlear implantation surgery [9]. Codex was included as part of the protocol of the EVATEM study for the detection of cognitive disorders amongst community-dwelling elderly people with memory complaints [10].

Despite the excellent metrics for dementia detection, Codex performance in detecting mild cognitive impairment (MCI), often a prodrome to dementia, is less certain. Ziso and Larner found that for a diagnosis of any cognitive impairment, dementia or MCI, Codex sensitivity was lower (0.68) whilst specificity was improved (0.91) compared to dementia detection [5,6]. In the EVATEM study (see Table 4 in [11]), Codex was found to have low sensitivity (0.32) but high specificity (0.85) for the detection of cognitive impairment (MCI and dementia, of which MCI patients made up a large majority, 176/182). These data suggest that Codex as originally formulated may be insufficiently sensitive for the detection of MCI.

We reasoned that minor modifications to the Codex decision tree might improve its screening utility for MCI. Specifically, since most MCI, whether of single or multiple domain type, includes an amnestic component, the use of a more stringent delayed recall paradigm might result in an instrument more sensitive to lesser degrees of cognitive impairment. Both the Montreal Cognitive Assessment (MoCA) [12] and the recently described Free-Cog (Professor Alistair Burns, Manchester, UK, personal communication, 2017) have a delayed recall test of five words rather than three words as in the MMSE [3]. Deriving a modified Codex from these instruments might therefore increase sensitivity for MCI, as shown in head to head studies of MoCA and MMSE [12,13], even allowing for the fewer spatial orientation components in these tests (MoCA 2, Free-Cog 3, versus MMSE 5).

We analysed data from pragmatic test accuracy studies of MoCA [14] and Free-Cog [15] and also reanalyzed data from a previous Codex test accuracy study [5,6] to examine whether a modified Codex might improve diagnostic utility for MCI.

2. Materials and Methods

Data from consecutive patient cohorts, referred to a dedicated cognitive function clinic based in secondary care and who were administered either MoCA (June 2015–May 2016 inclusive) [14] or Free-Cog (November 2017–October 2018 inclusive) [15], were analysed. Data from a previous consecutive patient cohort, referred to the same clinic and who were administered MMSE and sCDT (February–November 2012 inclusive) [5,6], were reanalysed. Standard diagnostic criteria for dementia (DSM-IV) and MCI [16] were used in these studies. Criterion diagnosis was by the judgment of an experienced clinician based on diagnostic criteria.

In the modified Codex decision tree derived from MoCA (Figure 1b), there were five delayed recall components but only two spatial orientation components [12], whereas in modified Codex derived from Free-Cog (Figure 1c), there were five delayed recall components but only three spatial orientation components. Both MoCA and Free-Cog incorporate clock drawing tests, unlike the MMSE, the scoring for which was simplified to 1 or 0 depending on whether or not all elements were completed correctly, as per the original Codex [1].

Categorical data were derived from the decision trees with differing probabilities of diagnosis (A = very low, B = low, C = high, D = very high), with categories C and D taken to be indicators of cognitive impairment [1]. Codex categories were not used in reference diagnosis to avoid review bias.

Dependent on the date of the study, either STARD or STARDdem guidelines for reporting diagnostic test accuracy studies in dementia [17,18] were observed. Standard summary measures of discrimination were calculated: sensitivity and specificity, false positive and false negative rates, Youden index (Y), positive and negative predictive values (PPV, NPV), predictive summary index (PSI), accuracy, net reclassification improvement (NRI), positive and negative likelihood ratios (LR+, LR−), diagnostic odds ratio (DOR), and clinical utility indexes (CUI+, CUI−). The recently described "likelihood to be diagnosed or misdiagnosed" (LDM) metric, the ratio of number needed to misdiagnose (NNM = 1/(1 − Accuracy)) to either number needed to diagnose (NND = 1/Y) or number needed to predict (NNP = 1/PSI), was also calculated; desirably, tests have LDM >1 [19].

3. Results

Baseline demographic data from the studies examining original Codex and modified Codex derived from MoCA or Free-Cog are shown in Table 1, along with the distribution of observed Codex categories versus diagnosis for each formulation of the decision tree (Figure 2).

Table 1. Study demographics and base category data.

Codex	N	Gender F:M (% Female)	Age Range (Median)	Diagnosis Dementia/MCI/SMC (%)	Codex Category A (%)	B (%)	C (%)	D (%)
Original	162	79:83 (49)	20–89 (61)	44/26/92 (27/16/57)	42 (25.9)	63 (38.8)	5 (3.1)	52 (32.1)
Modified from MoCA	257	116:141 (45)	22–89 (59)	43/75/139 (17/29/54)	15 (5.8)	159 (61.8)	9 (3.5)	74 (28.8)
Modified from Free-Cog	141	61:80 (43)	28–88 (62)	15/45/81 (11/32/57)	13 (9.2)	66 (46.8)	24 (17.0)	38 (26.9)

Abbreviations: MCI: mild cognitive impairment; SMC: subjective memory complaint; MoCA: Montreal Cognitive Assessment.

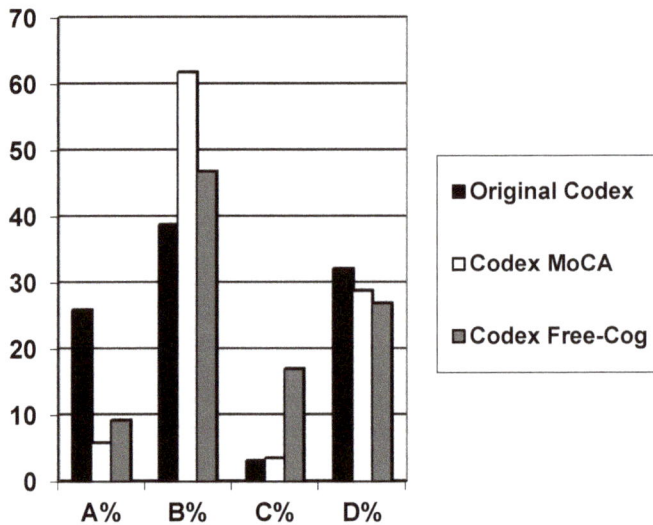

Figure 2. Codex categories versus patient diagnosis for each formulation of the decision tree; A = very low probability of dementia; B = low probability of dementia; C = high probability of dementia; D = very high probability of dementia (see Figure 1).

Measures of discrimination showed original Codex achieved very good sensitivity and specificity for the diagnosis of dementia versus no dementia, very good sensitivity for the diagnosis of dementia versus MCI, and very good specificity for the diagnosis of MCI versus no dementia (Table 2 and Figure 3a).

Table 2. Measures of discrimination for original Codex for the diagnosis of dementia and of MCI (with 95% confidence intervals).

	Diagnosis of Dementia vs. No Dementia (MCI + SMC)	Diagnosis of Dementia vs. MCI	Diagnosis of MCI vs. No Cognitive Impairment (SMC)
N	162 (44 vs. 118)	70 (44 vs. 26)	118 (26 vs. 92)
Prevalence (P = pre-test probability)	Dementia 0.27	Dementia 0.63	MCI 0.22
Pre-test odds (= P/1 − P)	Dementia 0.37	Dementia 1.69	MCI 0.28
Sensitivity (Se)	0.84 (0.73–0.95)	0.84 (0.73–0.95)	0.42 (0.23–0.61)
Specificity (Sp)	0.83 (0.76–0.90)	0.58 (0.39–0.77)	0.90 (0.84–0.96)
Y	0.67	0.42	0.32
PPV (= post-test probability)	0.65 (0.53–0.77)	0.77 (0.65–0.89)	0.55 (0.33–0.77)
NPV	0.93 (0.89–0.98)	0.68 (0.49–0.88)	0.85 (0.78–0.92)
PSI	0.58	0.45	0.40
Accuracy (Acc)	0.83 (0.78–0.89)	0.74 (0.64–0.85)	0.80 (0.72–0.87)
Net Reclassification Improvement (NRI = Acc − P)	0.56	0.11	0.58
LDM (= NNM/NND, NNM/NNP)	4.02, 3.48	1.63, 1.75	1.57, 1.97
LR+	4.96 (3.29–7.49) = moderate	1.99 (1.25–3.17) = slight	4.32 (2.01–9.30) = moderate
LR−	0.19 (0.13–0.29) = large	0.28 (0.17–0.44) = moderate	0.64 (0.30–1.38) = slight
DOR	25.9 (17.2–39.1)	7.21 (4.52–11.5)	6.76 (3.14–14.5)
Post-test odds (= pre-test odds × LR+)	Dementia 1.85	Dementia 3.36	MCI 1.21
CUI+ (= Se × PPV)	0.55 = adequate	0.65 = good	0.23 = very poor
CUI− (= Sp × NPV)	0.78 = good	0.39 = poor	0.76 = good

Abbreviations: MCI: mild cognitive impairment; SMC: subjective memory complaint; Y: Youden index; PPV: positive predictive value; NPV: negative predictive value; PSI: Predictive Summary Index; LDM: likelihood to diagnose or misdiagnose; NNM: number needed to misdiagnose; NND: number needed to diagnose; NNP: number needed to predict; LR+: positive likelihood ratio; LR−: negative likelihood ratio; DOR: diagnostic odds ratio; CUI+: positive clinical utility index; CUI−: negative clinical utility index.

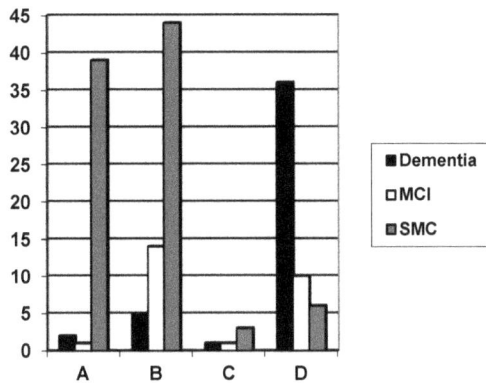

(a)

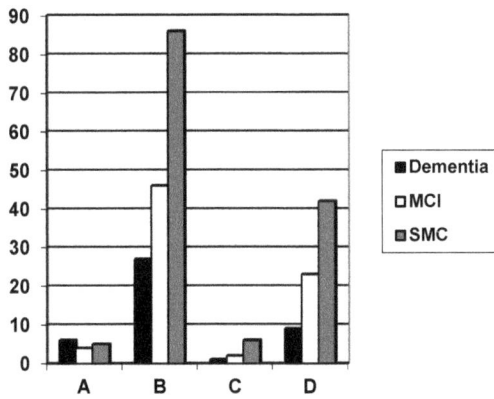

(b)

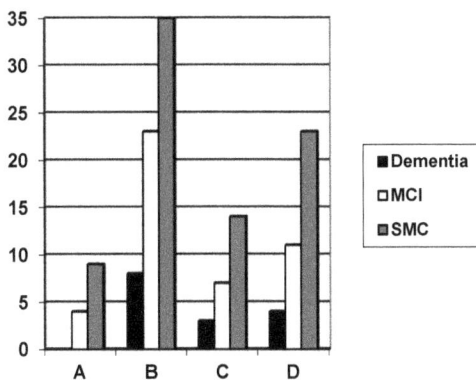

(c)

Figure 3. Diagnosis (dementia/MCI/SMC) plotted against: (**a**) Original Codex category (adapted from Ziso and Larner 2013 [5]); (**b**) Modified Codex category from MoCA; (**c**) Modified Codex category from Free-Cog; A = very low probability of dementia; B = low probability of dementia; C = high probability of dementia; D = very high probability of dementia (see Figure 1).

Measures of discrimination showed modified Codex derived from either MoCA (Table 3 and Figure 3b) or Free-Cog (Table 4 and Figure 3c) had lower sensitivity and specificity for both dementia and MCI diagnosis. For all parameters examined, original Codex performed better than either modified Codex.

Table 3. Measures of discrimination for modified Codex derived from MoCA for the diagnosis of dementia and of MCI (with 95% confidence intervals).

	Diagnosis of Dementia vs. No Dementia (MCI + SMC)	Diagnosis of Dementia vs. MCI	Diagnosis of MCI vs. No Cognitive Impairment (SMC)
N	257 (43 vs. 214)	118 (43 vs. 75)	214 (75 vs. 139)
Prevalence (P = pre-test probability)	Dementia 0.17	Dementia 0.36	MCI 0.35
Pre-test odds (= P/1 − P)	Dementia 0.20	Dementia 0.57	MCI 0.54
Sensitivity (Se)	0.23 (0.11–0.36)	0.23 (0.11–0.36)	0.33 (0.23–0.44)
Specificity (Sp)	0.66 (0.60–0.72)	0.67 (0.56–0.77)	0.65 (0.58–0.73)
Y	−0.11	−0.10	−0.02
PPV (= post-test probability)	0.12 (0.05–0.19)	0.29 (0.14–0.44)	0.34 (0.23–0.45)
NPV	0.81 (0.75–0.87)	0.60 (0.50–0.71)	0.65 (0.57–0.72)
PSI	−0.07	−0.11	−0.01
Accuracy (Acc)	0.59 (0.53–0.65)	0.51 (0.42–0.60)	0.54 (0.48–0.61)
Net Reclassification Improvement (NRI = Acc − P)	0.42	0.15	0.19
LDM (= NNM/NND, NNM/NNP)	−0.27, −0.17	−0.20, −0.22	−0.04, −0.02
LR+	0.68 (0.38–1.21) = slight	0.70 (0.37–1.31) = slight	0.97 (0.65–1.43) = slight
LR−	1.16 (0.66–2.07) = slight	1.15 (0.61–2.16) = slight	1.02 (0.69–1.51) = slight
DOR	0.59 (0.33–1.04)	0.61 (0.32–1.14)	0.95 (0.64–1.40)
Post-test odds (= pre-test odds × LR+)	Dementia 0.14	Dementia 0.40	MCI 0.52
CUI+ (= Se × PPV)	0.03 = very poor	0.07 = very poor	0.11 = very poor
CUI− (= Sp × NPV)	0.53 = adequate	0.40 = poor	0.42 = poor

Abbreviations: MCI: mild cognitive impairment; SMC: subjective memory complaint; Y: Youden index; PPV: positive predictive value; NPV: negative predictive value; PSI: Predictive Summary Index; LDM: likelihood to diagnose or misdiagnose; NNM: number needed to misdiagnose; NND: number needed to diagnose; NNP: number needed to predict; LR+: positive likelihood ratio; LR−: negative likelihood ratio; DOR: diagnostic odds ratio; CUI+: positive clinical utility index; CUI−: negative clinical utility index.

Table 4. Measures of discrimination for modified Codex derived from Free-Cog for the diagnosis of dementia and of MCI (with 95% confidence intervals).

	Diagnosis of Dementia vs. No Dementia (MCI + SMC)	Diagnosis of Dementia vs. MCI	Diagnosis of MCI vs. No Cognitive Impairment (SMC)
N	141 (15 vs. 126)	60 (15 vs. 45)	126 (45 vs. 81)
Prevalence (P = pre-test probability)	Dementia 0.11	Dementia 0.25	MCI 0.36
Pre-test odds (= P/1 − P)	Dementia 0.12	Dementia 0.33	MCI 0.56
Sensitivity (Se)	0.47 (0.21–0.72)	0.47 (0.21–0.72)	0.40 (0.26–0.54)
Specificity (Sp)	0.56 (0.48–0.65)	0.60 (0.47–0.74)	0.54 (0.43–0.65)
Y	0.03	0.07	−0.06
PPV (= post-test probability)	0.11 (0.03–0.19)	0.28 (0.10–0.46)	0.33 (0.20–0.45)
NPV	0.90 (0.83–0.97)	0.77 (0.63–0.91)	0.62 (0.51–0.73)
PSI	0.01	0.05	−0.05
Accuracy (Acc)	0.55 (0.47–0.64)	0.57 (0.44–0.69)	0.49 (0.40–0.58)
Net Reclassification Improvement (NRI = Acc − P)	0.44	0.32	0.13
LDM (= NNM/NND, NNM/NNP)	0.07, 0.02	0.63, 0.12	−0.12, −0.10
LR+	1.07 (0.60–1.91) = slight	1.17 (0.61–2.23) = slight	0.88 (0.57–1.35) = slight
LR−	0.95 (0.53–1.68) = slight	0.89 (0.46–1.70) = slight	1.10 (0.72–1.70) = slight
DOR	1.13 (0.63–2.01)	1.31 (0.69–2.51)	0.79 (0.52–1.22)
Post-test odds (= pre-test odds × LR+)	Dementia 0.13	Dementia 0.38	MCI 0.49
CUI+ (= Se × PPV)	0.05 = very poor	0.13 = very poor	0.13 = very poor
CUI− (= Sp × NPV)	0.51 = adequate	0.46 = poor	0.34 = very poor

Abbreviations: MCI: mild cognitive impairment; SMC: subjective memory complaint; Y: Youden index; PPV: positive predictive value; NPV: negative predictive value; PSI: Predictive Summary Index; LDM: likelihood to diagnose or misdiagnose; NNM: number needed to misdiagnose; NND: number needed to diagnose; NNP: number needed to predict; LR+: positive likelihood ratio; LR−: negative likelihood ratio; DOR: diagnostic odds ratio; CUI+: positive clinical utility index; CUI−: negative clinical utility index.

4. Discussion

The Codex decision tree proved easy to use, in both its original and modified forms. In particular, the ease of data extraction for modified Codex from both MoCA and Free-Cog required no extra sCDT step as required for original Codex derived from MMSE.

The performance of the original Codex for MCI diagnosis was very similar to that observed in the EVATEM study, namely, excellent specificity (0.90 vs. 0.85) and good NPV (0.85 vs 0.74) but poor sensitivity (0.42 vs 0.32) and modest PPV (0.55 vs 0.48). Original Codex therefore appears to be a test which is poor for ruling in a diagnosis of MCI.

The hope that minor modifications of the original Codex decision tree would afford better performance for MCI detection was not realized, with all parameters worse than for original Codex. Possible reasons for this failure might relate to the case mix in the various studies examined. There was an inversion in the frequency of dementia and MCI in the studies examining modified Codex compared to original Codex (see Table 1), reflecting changes in referral practice to the clinic. This changed the pretest odds of diagnosis in the different cohorts, specifically, in the latter cohorts examined with the modified forms of Codex, the pretest odds of MCI were higher than in the cohort administered original Codex. The typical shortcomings of clinic-based studies, such as the use of cross-sectional clinical diagnosis without delayed verification, are unlikely to explain the findings since this methodology was consistent between the study cohorts.

Many patients diagnosed clinically with subjective memory complaint were classified in category D (= very high probability of dementia) in the modified Codex decision trees (Figure 3b,c), hence false positives, suggesting inadequate test specificity. This might be anticipated if the modified Codex is, as hoped, more sensitive to cognitive impairment as a consequence of the changed (more stringent) delayed recall testing. However, some patients diagnosed clinically with dementia were nevertheless classified in category B (= low probability of dementia) in the modified Codex decision trees, hence false negatives, suggesting inadequate sensitivity. This might be a consequence of the changed (less stringent) spatial awareness testing.

Limitations of the study include the use of clinical diagnostic criteria for dementia and MCI, and the cross-sectional design which risks some miscategorisation of cases. The use of clinico-biological criteria incorporating imaging and CSF biomarkers [20] (not available to us) and longitudinal follow-up for the delayed verification of diagnosis might circumvent these problems. Moreover, "dementia" and "MCI" are broad categories which encompass a variety of neuropathological entities. Whilst Codex analysis by specific diagnosis might be desirable, this was not feasible with the small numbers of dementia and MCI cases (see Table 1). Furthermore, the goal of Codex, as for other cognitive screening instruments, is to identify those patients in whom additional testing is indicated to permit more fine-grained diagnostic classification. Screening tests can only screen for certain types of cognitive impairment related to dementia.

More broadly, this study poses questions about the value of decision trees and categorical data derived therefrom as opposed to the use of standard cognitive screening instruments (CSIs) generating quantitative data. Advantages of decision trees include the way in which they can facilitate medical decision making. The combination of choices from which the categories in a decision tree are derived may be taken to imply distinct management policies, hence in Codex, the categories A and B may result in patient reassurance, whilst categories C and D mandate further investigation, if necessary by onward referral to specialized services. However, medical decision-making policies may be less clear when using numerical cut-offs, although some CSIs, such as DemTect, further categorise cut-off scores in terms of suggested management policies [21]. In the future, the use of computerized techniques based on machine learning may provide better analyses than a decision tree [22,23].

The outcomes with modified Codex were less good than for the base tests (MoCA, Free-Cog), which generate quantitative data and from which Codex was extracted. The additional components in these CSIs may therefore add something which permits a more accurate diagnosis of MCI; data suggesting that CSI length (number of test items) correlates positively with measures of diagnostic accuracy have been presented [24]. Interestingly, in the EVATEM study, the best performance was found when all three tests examined (Codex, five-word test, and verbal fluency) were combined [11]. Whilst test brevity and the easy categorization of results is desirable in time-limited settings such as primary care, a different dispensation applies in dedicated cognitive disorders clinics based in secondary or tertiary care settings.

These data suggest that Codex, in either its original or modified form, is not sensitive for the diagnosis of MCI. Simple modifications of the decision tree which were anticipated to improve MCI detection did not produce the desired outcome, suggesting that tree impurity was not reduced, and that the modified tree was too shallow to identify MCI cases reliably. Hence, other instruments such as MoCA [12], MACE [14,25], and the Quick Mild Cognitive Impairment (Qmci) screen [26], some specifically designed for MCI identification, should be recommended for MCI diagnosis in preference to Codex.

5. Conclusions

Minor modifications to the Codex decision tree failed to improve diagnostic value, in particular sensitivity, for mild cognitive impairment.

Author Contributions: Data curation, A.J.L.; Formal analysis, A.J.L.; Investigation, B.Z. and A.J.L.; Methodology, B.Z. and A.J.L.; Project administration, B.Z.; Writing—original draft, A.J.L.; Writing—review & editing, B.Z. and A.J.L.

Funding: This research received no external funding.

Conflicts of Interest: The authors declare no conflict of interest.

References

1. Belmin, J.; Pariel-Madjlessi, S.; Surun, P.; Bentot, C.; Feteanu, D.; Lefebvre des Noettes, V.; Onen, F.; Drunat, O.; Trivalle, C.; Chassagne, P.; et al. The cognitive disorders examination (Codex) is a reliable 3-minute test for detection of dementia in the elderly (validation study in 323 subjects). *Presse Med.* **2007**, *36*, 1183–1190. [CrossRef] [PubMed]

2. Belmin, J.; Oasi, C.; Folio, P.; Pariel-Madjlessi, S. Codex, un test ultra-rapide pour le repérage des démences chez les sujets âgés. *Revue Geriatr.* **2007**, *32*, 627–631.

3. Folstein, M.F.; Folstein, S.E.; McHugh, P.R. "Mini-Mental State." A practical method for grading the cognitive state of patients for the clinician. *J. Psychiatr. Res.* **1975**, *12*, 189–198. [CrossRef]

4. Larner, A.J. Codex (cognitive disorders examination) for the detection of dementia and mild cognitive impairment. Codex pour la détection de la démence et du mild cognitive impairment. *Presse Med.* **2013**, *42*, e425–e428. [CrossRef] [PubMed]

5. Ziso, B.; Larner, A.J. Codex (cognitive disorders examination) for the detection of dementia and mild cognitive impairment: Diagnostic utility. *J. Neurol. Neurosurg. Psychiatry* **2013**, *84*, e2. [CrossRef]

6. Larner, A.J. *Dementia in Clinical Practice: A Neurological Perspective. Pragmatic Studies in the Cognitive Function Clinic*, 3rd ed.; Springer: London, UK, 2018; pp. 89–90.

7. Avgerinou, C.; Koufogianni, K.; Solini-Kosti, E.; Belmin, J. Validation of the Greek translation of the Cognitive Disorders Examination (Codex) for the detection of dementia in primary care. *Ann. Hellenic Med.* **2017**, *34*, 334–342.

8. Mézière, A.; Paillaud, E.; Belmin, J.; Pariel, S.; Herbaud, S.; Canouï-Poitrine, F.; Le Thuautd, A.; Martyce, J.; Plaud, B. Delirium in older people after proximal femoral fracture repair: role of a preoperative screening cognitive test. *Ann. Fr. Anesth. Reanim.* **2013**, *32*, e91–e96. [CrossRef]

9. Ambert-Dahan, E.; Routier, S.; Marot, L.; Bouccara, D.; Sterkers, O.; Ferrary, E.; Mosnier, I. Cognitive evaluation of cochlear implanted adults using CODEX and MoCA screening tests. *Otol. Neurotol.* **2017**, *38*, e282–e284. [CrossRef] [PubMed]

10. Vannier-Nitenberg, C.; Dauphinot, V.; Bongue, B.; Sass, C.; Rouch, I.; Beuachet, O.; Krolak-Salmon, P.; Fantino, B. Early detection of memory impairment in people over 65 years old consulting at Health Examination Centers for the French health insurance: the EVATEM protocol. *BMC Geriatr.* **2013**, *13*, 55. [CrossRef]

11. Vannier-Nitenberg, C.; Dauphinot, V.; Bongue, B.; Sass, C.; Bathsavanis, A.; Rouch, I.; Deville, N.; Beauchet, O.; Krolak-Salmon, P.; Fantino, B. Performance of cognitive tests, individually and combined, for the detection of cognitive disorders amongst community-dwelling elderly people with memory complaints: The EVATEM study. *Eur. J. Neurol.* **2016**, *23*, 554–561. [CrossRef]

12. Nasreddine, Z.S.; Phillips, N.A.; Bédirian, V.; Charbonneau, S.; Whitehead, V.; Collin, I.; Cummings, J.L.; Chertkow, H. The Montreal Cognitive Assessment, MoCA: A brief screening tool for mild cognitive impairment. *J. Am. Geriatr. Soc.* **2005**, *53*, 695–699. [CrossRef]

13. Larner, A.J. Comparing diagnostic accuracy of cognitive screening instruments: A weighted comparison approach. *Dement. Geriatr. Cogn. Disord. Extra* **2013**, *3*, 60–65. [CrossRef] [PubMed]

14. Larner, A.J. MACE versus MoCA: equivalence or superiority? Pragmatic diagnostic test accuracy study. *Int. Psychogeriatr.* **2017**, *29*, 931–937. [CrossRef] [PubMed]

15. Larner, A.J. Free-Cog: Pragmatic test accuracy study. *Dement. Geriatr. Cogn. Disord.* **2019**, *48*. accepted.

16. Winblad, B.; Palmer, K.; Kivipelto, M.; Jelic, V.; Fratiglioni, L.; Wahlund, L.-O.; Nordberg, A.; Bäckman, L.; Albert, M.; Almkvist, O.; et al. Mild cognitive impairment – beyond controversies, towards a consensus: report of the International Working Group on Mild Cognitive Impairment. *J. Intern. Med.* **2004**, *256*, 240–246. [CrossRef] [PubMed]

17. Bossuyt, P.M.; Reitsma, J.B.; Bruns, D.E.; Gatsonis, C.A.; Glasziou, P.P.; Irwig, L.M.; Moher, D.; Rennie, D.; de Vet, H.C.W.; Lijmer, J.G. The STARD statement for reporting studies of diagnostic accuracy: explanation and elaboration. *Clin. Chem.* **2003**, *49*, 7–18. [CrossRef]

18. Noel-Storr, A.H.; McCleery, J.M.; Richard, E.; Ritchie, C.W.; Flicker, L.; Cullum, S.J.; Davis, D.; Quinn, T.J.; Hyde, C.; Rutjes, A.W.; et al. Reporting standards for studies of diagnostic test accuracy in dementia: The STARDdem Initiative. *Neurology* **2014**, *83*, 364–373. [CrossRef] [PubMed]

19. Larner, A.J. Evaluating cognitive screening instruments with the "likelihood to be diagnosed or misdiagnosed" measure. *Int. J. Clin. Pract.* **2019**, *73*, e13265. [CrossRef]

20. Albert, M.S.; DeKosky, S.T.; Dickson, D.; Dubois, B.; Feldman, H.H.; Fox, N.C.; Gamst, A.; Holtzman, D.M.; Jagust, W.J.; Petersen, R.C.; et al. The diagnosis of mild cognitive impairment due to Alzheimer's disease: Recommendations from the National Institute on Aging-Alzheimer's Association workgroups on diagnostic guidelines for Alzheimer's disease. *Alzheimers Dement.* **2011**, *7*, 270–279. [CrossRef]

21. Kalbe, E.; Kessler, J. DemTect. In *Cognitive Screening Instruments. A Practical Approach*, 2nd ed.; Larner, A.J., Ed.; Springer: London, UK, 2017; pp. 197–208.

22. Pellegrini, E.; Ballerini, L.; Hernandez, M.D.C.V.; Chappell, F.M.; Gonzalez-Castro, V.; Anblagan, D.; Danso, S.; Muñoz-Maniega, S.; Job, D.; Pernet, C.; et al. Machine learning of neuroimaging for assisted diagnosis of cognitive impairment and dementia: A systematic review. *Alzheimers Dement. (Amst)* **2018**, *10*, 519–535. [CrossRef]

23. Chiu, P.Y.; Tang, H.; Wei, C.Y.; Zhang, C.; Hung, G.U.; Zhou, W. NMD-12: A new machine-learning derived screening instrument to detect mild cognitive impairment and dementia. *PLoS ONE* **2019**, *14*, e0213430. [CrossRef] [PubMed]

24. Larner, A.J. Performance-based cognitive screening instruments: an extended analysis of the time versus accuracy trade-off. *Diagnostics (Basel)* **2015**, *5*, 504–512. [CrossRef] [PubMed]

25. Hsieh, S.; McGrory, S.; Leslie, F.; Dawson, K.; Ahmed, S.; Butler, C.R.; Rowe, J.B.; Mioshi, E.; Hodges, J.R. The Mini-Addenbrooke's Cognitive Examination: A new assessment tool for dementia. *Dement. Geriatr. Cogn. Disord.* **2015**, *39*, 1–11. [CrossRef] [PubMed]

26. O'Caoimh, R.; Gao, Y.; McGlade, C.; Henry, L.; Gallagher, P.; Timmons, S.; Molloy, D.W. Comparison of the quick mild cognitive impairment (Qmci) screen and the SMMSE in screening for mild cognitive impairment. *Age Ageing* **2012**, *41*, 624–629. [CrossRef] [PubMed]

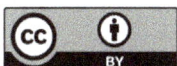

diagnostics

MDPI

Article

MACE for Diagnosis of Dementia and MCI: Examining Cut-Offs and Predictive Values

Andrew J. Larner

Cognitive Function Clinic, Walton Centre for Neurology and Neurosurgery, Liverpool L9 7LJ, UK;
a.larner@thewaltoncentre.nhs.uk or A.J.Larner@thewaltoncentre.nhs.uk

Received: 28 March 2019; Accepted: 1 May 2019; Published: 6 May 2019

Abstract: The definition of test cut-offs is a critical determinant of many paired and unitary measures of diagnostic or screening test accuracy, such as sensitivity and specificity, positive and negative predictive values, and correct classification accuracy. Revision of test cut-offs from those defined in index studies is frowned upon as a potential source of bias, seemingly accepting any biases present in the index study, for example related to sample bias. Data from a large pragmatic test accuracy study examining the Mini-Addenbrooke's Cognitive Examination (MACE) were interrogated to determine optimal test cut-offs for the diagnosis of dementia and mild cognitive impairment (MCI) using either the maximal Youden index or the maximal correct classification accuracy. Receiver operating characteristic (ROC) and precision recall (PR) curves for dementia and MCI were also plotted, and MACE predictive values across a range of disease prevalences were calculated. Optimal cut-offs were found to be a point lower than those defined in the index study. MACE had good metrics for the area under the ROC curve and for the effect size (Cohen's d) for both dementia and MCI diagnosis, but PR curves suggested the superiority for MCI diagnosis. MACE had high negative predictive value at all prevalences, suggesting that a MACE test score above either cut-off excludes dementia and MCI in any setting.

Keywords: diagnosis; dementia; mild cognitive impairment; Mini-Addenbrooke's Cognitive Examination

1. Introduction

The Mini-Addenbrooke's Cognitive Examination (MACE) is a shortened version of the Addenbrooke's Cognitive Examination-Revised (ACE-R) and ACE-III developed by Mokken scaling analysis of these longer instruments [1]. MACE comprises tests of attention, memory (7-item name and address), verbal fluency, clock drawing and memory recall (score range 0–30, impaired to normal), and takes between 5–10 min to administer.

In the index MACE study, two cut-off points were identified in the cohort examined ($n = 242$; Alzheimer's disease 28, behavioural variant frontotemporal dementia 23, primary progressive aphasia 82, corticobasal syndrome 21, controls 78): ≤25/30 had high sensitivity (0.85) and high specificity (0.87); and ≤21/30 had high specificity (1.00), and hence an abnormal score was almost certain to have come from a dementia patient. MACE was found to be more sensitive than the Mini-Mental State Examination (MMSE) and less likely to have ceiling effects [1].

The general applicability of these MACE cut-offs for the diagnosis of dementia and mild cognitive impairment (MCI) has not been widely examined. A Spanish translation administered to a cohort of mixed dementia patients and controls ($n = 175$) with relatively low educational experience found that a cut-off between 16/30 and 17/30 had optimal sensitivity (0.867) and specificity (0.870) for dementia diagnosis [2].

MACE was adopted in the author's practice, based in a dedicated Cognitive Function Clinic located at a regional neuroscience centre in the northwest United Kingdom in June 2014 [3], and has been routinely used since then. Access to a large dataset has provided the opportunity to examine a variety of parameters not hitherto examined. The aims of this study were:

- To determine optimal MACE cut-off points for the diagnosis of dementia and MCI, with the anticipation that cut-offs optimising sensitivity would also minimise false negative rate (FNR) and optimise negative predictive value (NPV) whilst cut-offs optimising specificity would minimise false positive rate (FPR) and optimise positive predictive value (PPV);
- To plot receiver operating characteristic (ROC) and precision recall (PR) curves for dementia and MCI, and to calculate areas under the ROC curves and Q* index (a measure of diagnostic value);
- To calculate MACE effect sizes (Cohen's d) for diagnosis of dementia and MCI;
- To calculate MACE predictive values across a range of disease prevalences.

2. Methods

Consecutive new patient referrals administered the MACE were included, seen over the period June 2014–December 2018 (inclusive), including data reported in previous studies [3–5]. Other than those with a pre-existing diagnosis of dementia, there were no exclusion criteria. As previously detailed [3–5], criterion diagnosis of dementia or mild cognitive impairment was by judgement of an experienced clinician using standard diagnostic criteria (DSM-IV; Petersen); in those without evidence of cognitive impairment, a diagnosis of subjective memory complaint (SMC) was made. MACE scores were not used to make criterion diagnoses to avoid review bias. Subjects gave informed consent, and the study protocol was approved by the institute's committee on human research.

MACE scores were plotted against diagnosis, and the Pearson 2 skewness coefficient (Sk2) was used to assess skew, where:

$$Sk2 = 3(\text{mean} - \text{median})/\text{standard deviation},$$

with values lying between –1 and +1 deemed acceptable for the elimination of floor or ceiling effects [6].

Various measures were calculated for all MACE cut-offs within the range deemed clinically sensible. Paired measures were: sensitivity (Sens, or recall) and specificity (Spec); positive and negative predictive values (PPV or precision, and NPV); positive and negative likelihood ratios (LR+ and LR–); and positive and negative clinical utility indexes (CUI+ and CUI–). Unitary or global measures were: correct classification accuracy (Acc); Youden index (Y, where Y = Sens + Spec – 1) [7]; predictive summary index (PSI, where PSI = PPV = NPV – 1) [8]; and identification index (II, where II = 2(Acc – 1) [9].

Two methods to optimise test cut-offs were examined [10,11], namely, maximising either Acc or Youden index.

In addition, various "number needed to" metrics were calculated: number needed to diagnose (NND, where NND = 1/Y); number needed to predict (NNP, where NNP = 1/PSI) [8]; and number needed to misdiagnose (NNM, where NNM = 1/(1 – Acc)) [12]. Also calculated were the "likelihood to be diagnosed or misdiagnosed" ratio (LDM, where LDM = NNM/NND or NNM/NNP) [13,14], and the "summary utility index" (SUI, where SUI = (CUI+ + CUI–)) [15]. The multiplicative inverse of the latter—the "number needed for screening utility" (NNSU = 1/SUI) [15]—was compared to the "number needed to screen" (NNS) metric, the multiplicative inverse of the "identification index" (II) [9], both rounded to the next highest integer value since they represent numbers of patients.

ROC curves were plotted (false positive rate versus sensitivity) and areas under the curve (AUC ROC) were calculated and categorised according to the scale of Metz [16]. The Q* index, a measure of diagnostic value [17], was determined as the point in ROC space where the anti-diagonal intersected the ROC curve (i.e., where Sens = Spec). Precision recall (PR) curves [18] were also plotted, as these have been recommended over ROC curves when analysing highly skewed datasets [19]. The F measure, or F1 score—the harmonic mean of precision and sensitivity—was also calculated as a global measure of accuracy [20].

Effect sizes (Cohen's d) were calculated as the difference of the means of diagnostic groups divided by the weighted pooled standard deviations of the groups [21]. Cohen's d values were categorised according to Sawilowsky's extension of Cohen's rules of thumb [22].

Predictive values across a range of disease prevalence (Prev) were calculated from observed sensitivity and specificity at the maximum Youden index for dementia and MCI, specifically at prevalence rates of 5%, 10%, 20% and 40% using the standard formulae:

$$PPV = Sens \times Prev/(Sens \times Prev) + [(1 - Spec) \times (1 - Prev)],$$

$$NPV = Spec \times (1 - Prev)/[Spec \times (1 - Prev)] + [(1 - Sens) \times Prev].$$

3. Results

A total of 755 patients were assessed with MACE (F:M = 352:403, 47% female; median age 60 years), of whom 114 were diagnosed with dementia (prevalence = 0.15) and 222 with MCI (prevalence = 0.29). The distribution of MACE scores by diagnosis, as seen in Figure 1, showed the anticipated unimodal negative skew (to the right, i.e., higher test scores = better performance). The Pearson 2 skewness coefficient (Sk2) was −0.48, suggesting that the population sampled was not from a normal distribution, although, as the value was between −1 and +1, the presence of floor or ceiling effects was probably excluded.

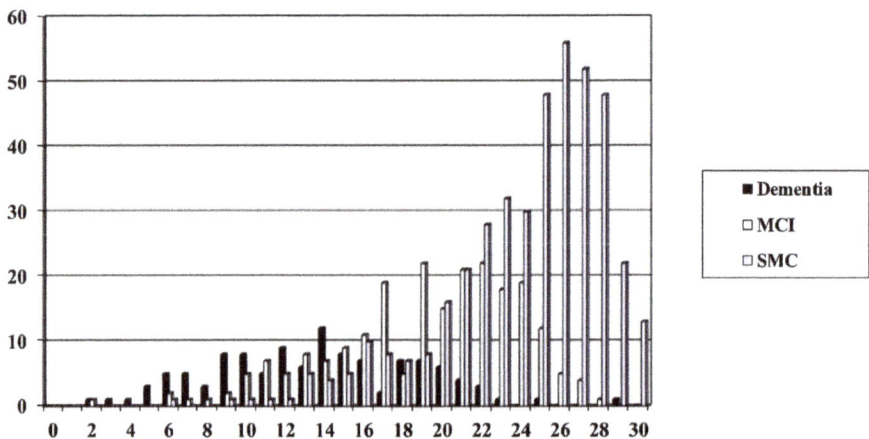

Figure 1. Mini-Addenbrooke's Cognitive Examination (MACE) scores versus patient diagnosis (*n* = 755). MCI: mild cognitive impairment; SMC: subjective memory complaint.

For the diagnosis of dementia (Tables 1 and 2), looking at all MACE cut-off values, the optimal cut-off determined by maximal Youden index was ≤20/30 (sensitivity 0.91, specificity 0.71). By maximal correct classification accuracy the optimal cut-off was ≤14/30 (sensitivity 0.59, specificity 0.92). This latter cut-off also had the maximal values of PSI and LDM (Table 3), the latter also found at ≤15/30, which was also the cut-off for the maximal value of SUI and F measure.

For the diagnosis of MCI (Tables 4 and 5), looking at all MACE cut-off values, the optimal cut-off determined by maximal Youden index was ≤24/30 (sensitivity 0.90, specificity 0.57). By maximal correct classification accuracy the optimal cut-off was ≤19/30 (sensitivity 0.47, specificity 0.88). Both cut-offs coincided with the maximal values of LDM (Table 6), whereas maximum PSI and F measure were at the same cut-off as maximal Youden index (cf. diagnosis of dementia), whilst maximal SUI was at ≤22/30 and ≤21/30.

Table 1. Diagnosis of dementia: paired measures of discrimination at various MACE cut-offs.

Cut-off	Sensitivity (= Recall); Specificity	False Positive Rate (FPR); False Negative Rate (FNR)	PPV (= Precision); NPV	LR+; LR−	CUI+; CUI−
≤29/30	1.00; 0.02	0.98; 0	0.15; 1.00	1.02; 0	0.15; 0.02
≤28/30	0.99; 0.06	0.94; 0.01	0.16; 0.97	1.05; 0.16	0.16; 0.05
≤27/30	0.99; 0.13	0.87; 0.01	0.17; 0.99	1.14; 0.07	0.17; 0.13
≤26/30	0.99; 0.22	0.78; 0.01	0.18; 0.99	1.27; 0.04	0.18; 0.22
≤25/30 *	0.99; 0.32	0.68; 0.01	0.20; 0.99	1.45; 0.03	0.20; 0.32
≤24/30	0.98; 0.41	0.59; 0.02	0.23; 0.99	1.66; 0.04	0.23; 0.41
≤23/30	0.98; 0.49	0.51; 0.02	0.25; 0.99	1.91; 0.04	0.25; 0.49
≤22/30	0.97; 0.56	0.44; 0.03	0.28; 0.99	2.23; 0.05	0.27; 0.55
≤21/30 *	0.95; 0.64	0.36; 0.05	0.32; 0.99	2.64; 0.08	0.30; 0.63
≤20/30	0.91; 0.71	0.29; 0.09	0.36; 0.98	3.11; 0.12	0.33; 0.70
≤19/30	0.86; 0.76	0.24; 0.14	0.38; 0.97	3.51; 0.19	0.33; 0.74
≤18/30	0.80; 0.80	0.20; 0.20	0.42; 0.96	4.03; 0.25	0.34; 0.77
≤17/30	0.74; 0.82	0.18; 0.26	0.42; 0.95	4.11; 0.32	0.31; 0.78
≤16/30	0.72; 0.86	0.14; 0.28	0.48; 0.95	5.24; 0.33	0.35; 0.82
≤15/30	0.66; 0.90	0.10; 0.34	0.53; 0.94	6.29; 0.38	0.35; 0.85
≤14/30	0.59; 0.92	0.08; 0.41	0.56; 0.93	7.11; 0.45	0.33; 0.86
≤13/30	0.48; 0.93	0.07; 0.52	0.57; 0.91	7.36; 0.55	0.27; 0.85

CUI+ and CUI−: positive and negative clinical utility indices; LR+ and LR−: positive and negative likelihood ratios; NPV: negative predictive value; PPV: positive predictive value. * Test cut-off established in index study (Hsieh et al. 2015 [1]).

Table 2. Diagnosis of dementia: unitary measures of discrimination at various MACE cut-offs.

Cut-off	Acc; Inacc	Y (= Sens + Spec − 1)	PSI (= PPV + NPV − 1)	II (= 2(Acc − 1))	DOR (= LR+/LR−)	SUI (= CUI+ + CUI−)	F Measure (F1 Score)
≤29/30	0.17; 0.83	0.02	0.15	−0.66	∞	0.15	0.27
≤28/30	0.20; 0.80	0.05	0.13	−0.61	6.72	0.21	0.27
≤27/30	0.26; 0.74	0.12	0.16	−0.48	17.3	0.30	0.29
≤26/30	0.37; 0.63	0.21	0.17	−0.33	31.9	0.40	0.31
≤25/30 *	0.42; 0.58	0.31	0.19	−0.17	52.0	0.52	0.34
≤24/30	0.49; 0.51	0.39	0.22	−0.01	38.7	0.64	0.37
≤23/30	0.56; 0.44	0.47	0.24	0.12	52.8	0.74	0.40
≤22/30	0.63; 0.37	0.53	0.27	0.25	47.7	0.82	0.44
≤21/30 *	0.69; 0.31	0.59	0.31	0.37	32.2	0.93	0.48
≤20/30	0.74; 0.26	0.619	0.34	0.48	25.1	1.03	0.51
≤19/30	0.77; 0.23	0.614	0.35	0.54	18.9	1.07	0.53
≤18/30	0.80; 0.20	0.60	0.38	0.60	16.0	1.11	0.55
≤17/30	0.81; 0.19	0.56	0.37	0.62	12.8	1.09	0.54
≤16/30	0.84; 0.16	0.58	0.43	0.68	16.1	1.17	0.58
≤15/30	0.859; 0.14	0.56	0.46	0.72	16.5	1.20	0.59
≤14/30	0.867; 0.13	0.51	0.49	0.74	15.8	1.19	0.57
≤13/30	0.866; 0.13	0.41	0.49	0.73	13.3	1.12	0.52

Acc: correct classification accuracy; DOR: diagnostic odds ratio; II: identification index; Inacc: inaccuracy; PSI: predictive summary index; Sens: sensitivity; Spec: specificity; SUI: summary utility index; Y: Youden index. * Test cut-off established in index study (Hsieh et al. 2015 [1]).

Table 3. Diagnosis of dementia: "number needed to" measures (rounded to next highest integer value) and "likelihood to be diagnosed or misdiagnosed" at various MACE cut-offs.

Cut-off	NND (= 1/Y)	NNP (= 1/PSI)	NNM (= 1/Inacc)	NNS (= 1/II)	NNSU (= 1/SUI)	LDM (= NNM/NND; NNM/NNP)
≤29/30	50	7	2	−2	7	0.04; 0.29
≤28/30	20	8	2	−2	5	0.10; 0.25
≤27/30	9	7	2	−3	4	0.22; 0.29
≤26/30	5	6	2	−4	3	0.40; 0.33
≤25/30 *	4	6	2	−7	2	0.50; 0.33
≤24/30	3	5	2	−108	2	0.67; 0.40
≤23/30	3	5	3	9	2	1.00; 0.60
≤22/30	2	4	3	4	2	1.50; 0.75
≤21/30 *	2	4	4	3	2	2.00; 1.00
≤20/30	2	3	4	3	1	2.00; 1.33
≤19/30	2	3	5	2	1	2.50; 1.67
≤18/30	2	3	5	2	1	2.50; 1.67
≤17/30	2	3	6	2	1	3.00; 2.00
≤16/30	2	3	7	2	1	3.50; 2.33
≤15/30	2	3	8	2	1	4.00; 2.67
≤14/30	2	3	8	2	1	4.00; 2.67
≤13/30	3	3	8	2	1	2.67; 2.67

LDM: likelihood to diagnose or misdiagnose; NND: number needed to diagnose; NNM: number needed to misdiagnose; NNP: number needed to predict; NNS: number needed to screen; NNSU: number needed for screening utility. * Test cut-off established in index study (Hsieh et al. 2015 [1]).

Table 4. Diagnosis of MCI: paired measures of discrimination at various MACE cut-offs.

Cut-off	Sensitivity (= Recall); Specificity	False Positive (FPR); False Negative (FNR)	PPV (= Precision); NPV	LR+; LR−	CUI+; CUI−
≤29/30	1.00; 0.03	0.97; 0	0.35; 1.00	1.03; 0	0.35; 0.03
≤28/30	1.00; 0.09	0.91, 0	0.37; 1.00	1.09; 0	0.37; 0.09
≤27/30	0.99; 0.20	0.80; 0.01	0.40; 0.99	1.25; 0.02	0.40; 0.20
≤26/30	0.98; 0.32	0.68; 0.02	0.43; 0.96	1.45; 0.07	0.42; 0.31
≤25/30 *	0.95; 0.46	0.54; 0.05	0.48; 0.95	1.76; 0.10	0.46; 0.44
≤24/30	0.90; 0.57	0.43; 0.10	0.53; 0.92	2.11; 0.17	0.48; 0.52
≤23/30	0.82; 0.64	0.36; 0.18	0.55; 0.87	2.29; 0.29	0.45; 0.56
≤22/30	0.73; 0.72	0.28; 0.27	0.58; 0.84	2.63; 0.37	0.42; 0.60
≤21/30 *	0.64; 0.79	0.21; 0.36	0.61; 0.80	2.99; 0.46	0.39; 0.63
≤20/30	0.54; 0.84	0.16; 0.46	0.63; 0.77	3.33; 0.55	0.34; 0.65
≤19/30	0.47; 0.88	0.12; 0.53	0.67; 0.76	3.81; 0.60	0.31; 0.67
≤18/30	0.37; 0.89	0.11; 0.63	0.65; 0.73	3.56; 0.70	0.24; 0.65

LR+; LR− = positive and negative likelihood ratio; CUI+; CUI− = positive and negative clinical utility index. * = test cut-off established in index study (Hsieh et al. 2015 [1]).

Table 5. Diagnosis of MCI: unitary measures of discrimination at various MACE cut-offs.

Cut-off	Acc; Inacc	Y (= Sens + Spec − 1)	PSI (= PPV + NPV − 1)	II (= 2(Acc − 1))	DOR (= LR+/LR−)	SUI (= CUI+ + CUI−)	F Measure (F1 Score)
≤29/30	0.37; 0.63	0.03	0.35	−0.26	∞	0.38	0.52
≤28/30	0.40; 0.60	0.09	0.37	−0.20	∞	0.46	0.54
≤27/30	0.48; 0.52	0.19	0.39	−0.05	55.4	0.60	0.57
≤26/30	0.55; 0.45	0.30	0.39	0.10	20.9	0.73	0.60
≤25/30 *	0.63; 0.37	0.41	0.43	0.26	17.9	0.90	0.64
≤24/30	0.69; 0.31	0.47	0.45	0.37	12.2	1.00	0.67
≤23/30	0.70; 0.30	0.46	0.42	0.41	8.00	1.01	0.66
≤22/30	0.73; 0.27	0.45	0.42	0.45	7.13	1.02	0.65
≤21/30*	0.73; 0.27	0.43	0.41	0.47	6.45	1.02	0.62
≤20/30	0.73; 0.27	0.38	0.40	0.47	6.07	0.99	0.58
≤19/30	0.74; 0.26	0.35	0.43	0.47	6.33	0.98	0.55
≤18/30	0.71; 0.29	0.26	0.38	0.43	5.09	0.89	0.48

Acc: correct classification accuracy; DOR: diagnostic odds ratio; II: identification index; Inacc: inaccuracy; PSI: predictive summary index; SUI: summary utility index; Y: Youden index. * Test cut-off established in index study (Hsieh et al. 2015 [1]).

Table 6. Diagnosis of MCI: "number needed to" measures (rounded to next highest integer value) and "likelihood to be diagnosed or misdiagnosed" at various MACE cut-offs.

Cut-off	NND (= 1/Y)	NNP (= 1/PSI)	NNM (= 1/Inaccuracy)	NNS (= 1/II)	NNSU (= 1/SUI)	LDM (= NNM/NND; NNM/NNP)
≤29/30	34	3	2	−4	3	0.06; 0.67
≤28/30	12	3	2	−6	3	0.17; 0.67
≤27/30	6	3	2	−21	2	0.33; 0.67
≤26/30	4	3	3	10	2	0.75; 1.00
≤25/30 *	3	3	3	4	2	1.00; 1.00
≤24/30	3	3	4	3	1	1.33; 1.33
≤23/30	3	3	4	3	1	1.33; 1.33
≤22/30	3	3	4	3	1	1.33; 1.33
≤21/30 *	3	3	4	3	1	1.33; 1.33
≤20/30	3	3	4	3	2	1.33; 1.33
≤19/30	3	3	4	3	2	1.33; 1.33
≤18/30	4	3	4	3	2	1.00; 1.33

LDM: likelihood to diagnose or misdiagnose; NND: number needed to diagnose; NNM: number needed to misdiagnose; NNP: number needed to predict; NNS: number needed to screen; NNSU: number needed for screening utility. * Test cut-off established in index study (Hsieh et al. 2015 [1]).

Comparison of the values for NNS and NNSU (Tables 3 and 6) showed negative values of NNS (which are clinically meaningless) when identification index (II) had negative values, but this was not the case with NNSU, since by definition SUI cannot be <0.

A ROC curve was plotted for the diagnosis of dementia and MCI (Figure 2). The AUC ROC was 0.89 (95% confidence interval (CI) 0.86–0.92) for the diagnosis of dementia and 0.81 (95% CI 0.77–0.84) for the diagnosis of MCI, hence the AUC ROC values were categorised as good [16] for the diagnosis of both dementia vs. no dementia and MCI vs. SMC. The Q* index for dementia was 0.8 (comparable to the value of 0.76 found in a previous study examining the first 135 patients in this cohort [3]) and for MCI it was 0.73. PR curves (Figure 3) did not show the desired approximation to the top-right corner of the graph, reflecting the relatively poor PPV of MACE, but did show greater area under the curve for MCI versus dementia.

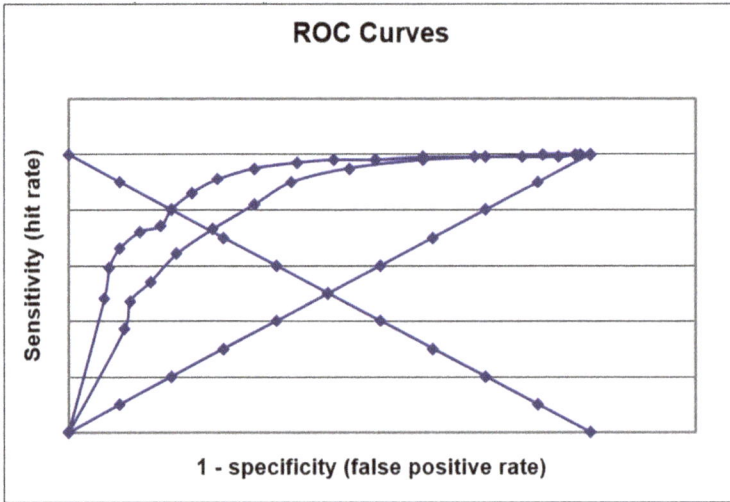

Figure 2. MACE receiver operating characteristic (ROC) plots for the diagnosis of dementia (upper; area under the curve (AUC) = 0.89) and MCI (lower; AUC = 0.81) with chance diagonal ($y = x$) and anti-diagonal ($y = 1 - x$) lines.

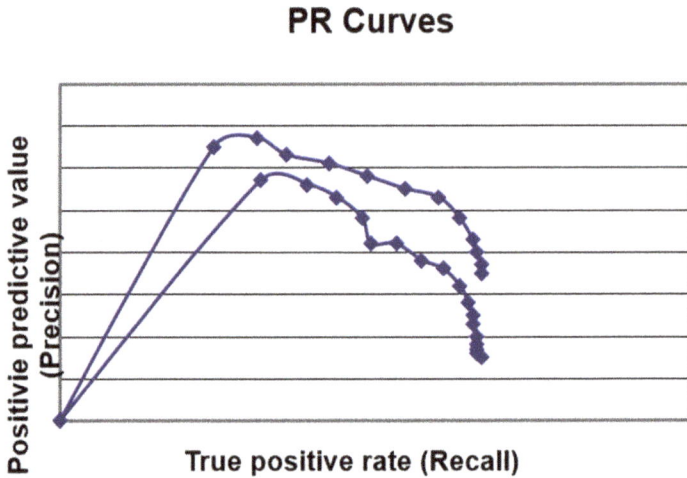

Figure 3. MACE precision recall (PR) curves for the diagnosis of dementia (lower) and MCI (upper); note the reversal of position versus ROC curves.

Effect sizes (Cohen's d) were 1.74 for dementia and 1.13 for MCI, hence very large and large, respectively [22].

PPV and NPV for MACE calculated at prevalence rates of 5%, 10%, 20% and 40% using the sensitivity and specificity figures at the maximum Youden index showed high NPV (≥0.9) at all prevalences examined, but with less-impressive figures for PPV, optimal at higher disease prevalences (Table 7).

Table 7. MACE predictive values at differing disease prevalence of dementia and MCI (0.05–0.4).

	Prevalence					
	0.05	0.1	0.15 (Observed)	0.2	0.29 (Observed)	0.4
PPV dementia (cut-off ≤20/30)	0.14	0.26	0.36	0.44	-	0.68
NPV dementia (cut-off ≤20/30)	0.99	0.99	0.98	0.97	-	0.92
PPV MCI (cut-off ≤24/30)	0.10	0.19	-	0.34	0.53	0.58
NPV MCI (cut-off ≤24/30)	0.99	0.98	-	0.96	0.92	0.90

4. Discussion

This study of a large cohort of patients examined with the Mini-Addenbrooke's Cognitive Examination suggested that the optimal test cut-offs differ slightly from those suggested in the index study, being a point lower for both high-sensitivity (≤24/30 vs. ≤25/30) and high-specificity (≤20/30 vs. ≤21/30) cut-offs. Even allowing for the objections raised to changing test cut-offs because of risk of bias [23], these findings suggest a possible need for cut-off revision when using MACE in general cognitive clinics, as well as for patient educational level [2].

ROC curves suggested that MACE had adequate accuracy for the diagnosis of dementia and MCI—a finding corroborated by the measure of effect size (Cohen's d). The Q* index for dementia (0.80) was comparable to that found for other cognitive screening instruments [24], but the Q* index for MCI was lower (0.73). However, PR curves suggested better MACE performance (i.e., distinguishable classification performance) for the diagnosis of MCI than for dementia, consistent with findings in previous comparative studies of MACE with the Montreal Cognitive Assessment (MoCA)—a test designed specifically for MCI diagnosis (equivalent MACE performance) [25,26], and Free-Cog (superior MACE performance) [5]. The use of PR curves [18] in diagnostic test accuracy studies is worth emphasizing (to the author's knowledge this is the first such use for dementia test accuracy studies), since these avoid some of the "optimism" of ROC curves (resulting from their combining test accuracy over a range of thresholds which may be both clinically relevant and clinically nonsensical) [27]. PR curves are more informative than ROC curves for skewed datasets [19]. Area under the PR curve may be calculated, although this is not straightforward [28], and visual interpretation may be adequate to denote better classification performance (as for ROC curves).

The comparison of NNS [9] and NNSU [15] in this study was also instructive, demonstrating some of the difficulties in working with reciprocals (multiplicative inverses). By definition, the identification index (II) ranges from −1 to +1, and hence NNS ranges from −∞ to +∞ [9]. As II approaches 0, values of NNS are inflated (e.g., Table 3, cut-off ≤24/30; Table 6, cut-off ≤27/30), and when II is negative then NNS also has a negative value. The latter finding is problematic from the clinical standpoint: "number needed to" metrics were originally designed to appeal intuitively at the individual level, so negative values (representing non-individuals?) are meaningless. The construction of SUI is such that by definition its range is from 0 to 2, and hence NNSU ranges from ∞ (no screening value) to 0.5 (perfect screening utility) [15], avoiding the problems encountered with II and NNS.

The high NPV (≥0.9) at all disease prevalences examined (0.05 to 0.4) suggests that a MACE test score above either cut-off excludes dementia and MCI in any setting. PPV was less impressive, but improved with increasing disease prevalence, suggesting a case-finding role for MACE in dedicated cognitive and memory clinics.

In summary, in addition to being quick, easy to use and score and acceptable to patients [1,3,4], when using appropriate cut-offs MACE is a sensitive test for the identification of cognitive impairment and for excluding dementia and MCI with scores below the cut-offs.

Diagnostics **2019**, *9*, 51

Funding: This research received no external funding.

Acknowledgments: Nil.

Conflicts of Interest: The author declares no conflict of interest.

References

1. Hsieh, S.; McGrory, S.; Leslie, F.; Dawson, K.; Ahmed, S.; Butler, C.R.; Rowe, J.B.; · Mioshi, E.; · Hodges, J.R. The Mini-Addenbrooke's Cognitive Examination: A new assessment tool for dementia. *Dement. Geriatr. Cogn. Disord.* **2015**, *39*, 1–11. [CrossRef] [PubMed]
2. Matias-Guiu, J.A.; Fernandez-Bobadilla, R. Validation of the Spanish-language version of Mini-Addenbrooke's Cognitive Examination as a dementia screening tool [in Spanish]. *Neurologia* **2016**, *31*, 646–648. [CrossRef] [PubMed]
3. Larner, A.J. Mini-Addenbrooke's Cognitive Examination: A pragmatic diagnostic accuracy study. *Int. J. Geriatr. Psychiatry* **2015**, *30*, 547–548. [CrossRef] [PubMed]
4. Williamson, J.C.; Larner, A.J. MACE for diagnosis of dementia and MCI: 3-year pragmatic diagnostic test accuracy study. *Dement. Geriatr. Cogn. Disord.* **2018**, *45*, 300–307. [CrossRef] [PubMed]
5. Larner, A.J. Free-Cog: Pragmatic test accuracy study. *Dement. Geriatr. Cogn. Disord.* **2019**, *48*. accepted.
6. Doane, D.P.; Seward, L.E. Measuring skewness: A forgotten statistic? *J. Stat. Educ.* **2011**, *19*, 1–18. [CrossRef]
7. Youden, W.J. Index for rating diagnostic tests. *Cancer* **1950**, *3*, 32–35. [CrossRef]
8. Linn, S.; Grunau, P.D. New patient-oriented summary measure of net total gain in certainty for dichotomous diagnostic tests. *Epidemiol. Perspect. Innov.* **2006**, *3*, 11. [CrossRef] [PubMed]
9. Mitchell, A.J. Index test. In *Encyclopedia of Medical Decision Making*; Kattan, M.W., Ed.; Sage: Los Angeles, CA, USA, 2009; pp. 613–617.
10. Larner, A.J. Optimizing the cutoffs of cognitive screening instruments in pragmatic diagnostic accuracy studies: Maximising accuracy or Youden index? *Dement. Geriatr. Cogn. Disord.* **2015**, *39*, 167–175. [CrossRef] [PubMed]
11. O'Caoimh, R.; Gao, Y.; Svendovski, A.; Gallagher, P.; Eustace, J.; Molloy, D.W. Comparing approaches to optimize cut-off scores for short cognitive screening instruments in mild cognitive impairment and dementia. *J. Alzheimers Dis.* **2017**, *57*, 123–133. [CrossRef] [PubMed]
12. Habibzadeh, F.; Yadollahie, M. Number needed to misdiagnose: A measure of diagnostic test effectiveness. *Epidemiology* **2013**, *24*, 170. [CrossRef] [PubMed]
13. Larner, A.J. Number needed to diagnose, predict, or misdiagnose: Useful metrics for non-canonical signs of cognitive status? *Dement. Geriatr. Cogn. Dis. Extra* **2018**, *8*, 321–327. [CrossRef] [PubMed]
14. Larner, A.J. Evaluating cognitive screening instruments with the "likelihood to be diagnosed or misdiagnosed" measure. *Int. J. Clin. Pract.* **2019**, *73*, e13265. [CrossRef]
15. Larner, A.J. *Manual of Screeners for Dementia: Pragmatic Test Accuracy Studies*; Springer: London, UK, 2019, in press.
16. Metz, C.E. Basic principles of ROC analysis. *Semin. Nucl. Med.* **1978**, *8*, 283–298. [CrossRef]
17. Walter, S.D. Properties of the summary receiver operating characteristic (SROC) curve for diagnostic test data. *Stat. Med.* **2002**, *21*, 1237–1256. [CrossRef]
18. Davis, J.; Goadrich, M. The relationship between Precision-Recall and ROC curves. In *ICML '06: Proceedings of the 23rd International Conference on Machine Learning*; ACM: New York, NY, USA, 2006; pp. 233–240.
19. Saito, T.; Rehmsmeier, M. The precision-recall plot is more informative than the ROC plot when evaluating binary classifiers on imbalanced datasets. *PLoS ONE* **2015**, *10*, e0118432. [CrossRef]
20. Powers, D.M.W. Evaluation: From precision, recall and F-measure to ROC, informedness, markedness and correlation. *J. Mach. Learn. Technol.* **2011**, *2*, 37–63.
21. Cohen, J. *Statistical Power Analysis for the Behavioral Sciences*, 2nd ed.; Lawrence Erlbaum: Hillsdale, NJ, USA, 1988.
22. Sawilowsky, S.S. New effect sizes rules of thumb. *J. Mod. Appl. Stat. Methods* **2009**, *8*, 597–599. [CrossRef]
23. Davis, D.H.; Creavin, S.T.; Noel-Storr, A.; Quinn, T.J.; Smailagic, N.; Hyde, C.; Brayne, C.; McShane, R.; Cullum, S. Neuropsychological tests for the diagnosis of Alzheimer's disease dementia and other dementias: A generic protocol for cross-sectional and delayed-verification studies. *Cochrane Database Syst. Rev.* **2013**, *3*, CD010460. [CrossRef]

24. Larner, A.J. The Q* index: A useful global measure of dementia screening test accuracy? *Dement. Geriatr. Cogn. Dis. Extra* **2015**, *5*, 265–270. [CrossRef]

25. Nasreddine, Z.S.; Phillips, N.A.; Bédirian, V.; Charbonneau, S.; Whitehead, V.; Collin, I.; Cummings, J.L.; Chertkow, H. The Montreal Cognitive Assessment, MoCA: A brief screening tool for mild cognitive impairment. *J. Am. Geriatr. Soc.* **2005**, *53*, 695–699. [CrossRef] [PubMed]

26. Larner, A.J. MACE versus MoCA: equivalence or superiority? Pragmatic diagnostic test accuracy study. *Int. Psychogeriatr.* **2017**, *29*, 931–937. [CrossRef] [PubMed]

27. Ozenne, B.; Subtil, F.; Maucort-Boulch, D. The precision-recall curve overcame the optimism of the receiver operating characteristic curve in rare diseases. *J. Clin. Epidemiol.* **2015**, *68*, 855–859. [CrossRef] [PubMed]

28. Keilwagen, J.; Grosse, I.; Grau, J. Area under precision-recall curves for weighted and unweighted data. *PLoS ONE* **2014**, *9*, e92209. [CrossRef] [PubMed]

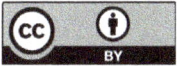

diagnostics

MDPI

Article

Comparing the Diagnostic Accuracy of Two Cognitive Screening Instruments in Different Dementia Subtypes and Clinical Depression

Rónán O'Caoimh [1,2,*] and D. William Molloy [1]

[1]   Centre for Gerontology and Rehabilitation, University College Cork, St Finbarr's Hospital, Douglas road,
     T12 XH60 Cork City, Ireland
[2]   Department of Geriatric Medicine, Mercy University Hospital, Grenville Place, T12 WE28 Cork City, Ireland
*   Correspondence: rocaoimh@hotmail.com or rocaoimh@muh.ie

Received: 1 July 2019; Accepted: 6 August 2019; Published: 8 August 2019

Abstract: Short but accurate cognitive screening instruments are required in busy clinical practice. Although widely-used, the diagnostic accuracy of the standardised Mini-Mental State Examination (SMMSE) in different dementia subtypes remains poorly characterised. We compared the SMMSE to the Quick Mild Cognitive Impairment (Q*mci*) screen in patients (*n* = 3020) pooled from three memory clinic databases in Canada including those with mild cognitive impairment (MCI) and Alzheimer's, vascular, mixed, frontotemporal, Lewy Body and Parkinson's dementia, with and without co-morbid depression. Caregivers (*n* = 875) without cognitive symptoms were included as normal controls. The median age of patients was 77 (Interquartile = ±9) years. Both instruments accurately differentiated cognitive impairment (MCI or dementia) from controls. The SMMSE most accurately differentiated Alzheimer's (AUC 0.94) and Lewy Body dementia (AUC 0.94) and least accurately identified MCI (AUC 0.73), vascular (AUC 0.74), and Parkinson's dementia (AUC 0.81). The Q*mci* had statistically similar or greater accuracy in distinguishing all dementia subtypes but particularly MCI (AUC 0.85). Co-morbid depression affected accuracy in those with MCI. The SMMSE and Q*mci* have good-excellent accuracy in established dementia. The SMMSE is less suitable in MCI, vascular and Parkinson's dementia, where alternatives including the Q*mci* screen may be used. The influence of co-morbid depression on scores merits further investigation.

Keywords: dementia; mild cognitive impairment; screening; accuracy; standardised mini-mental state examination; quick mild cognitive impairment screen

1. Introduction

Although short cognitive screening instruments (CSIs) such as the Mini-Mental State Examination (MMSE) [1] and its standardised version, the SMMSE [2,3] are widely used in clinical practice and research studies, their accuracy and hence suitability for use in detecting different dementia subtypes is poorly characterised [4]. Numerous studies including recent systematic reviews show that the MMSE has poor accuracy and that an alternative instrument should be used to identify those with mild cognitive impairment (MCI) [5], a prodromal state characterised by cognitive deficits without loss of social or occupation function and before the onset of dementia [6]. Other instruments such as the Memory Alteration Test [7], the Quick Mild Cognitive Impairment (Q*mci*) screen [8] and Montreal Cognitive Assessment (MoCA) [9] are recommended as alternatives [5,10]. The MMSE has a "floor" effect such that a score of zero does not always support dementia and a "low ceiling" effect such that a normal score does not always mean normal cognition [11]. It is also influenced by age and education meaning that it is poorly sensitive when used among older and less educated adults [12,13]. It also has poor reliability, which led to the development of the SMMSE. Despite these issues, the MMSE remains the most widely used CSI in clinical practice [14].

Given that the MMSE and SMMSE cover a limited number of cognitive domains [2,3], their diagnostic accuracy in different types of dementia is unclear. The SMMSE lacks a subtest measuring executive function, which suggests that it is less useful in those with Parkinson's disease cognitive impairment [15] and is overly weighted towards language skills, making it less useful in frontotemporal dementia [16]. Compared with other short CSIs such as the MoCA, the MMSE has poor accuracy in detecting vascular cognitive impairment, which is often characterised by impaired attention, executive and visuospatial dysfunction, all poorly assessed with the MMSE subtests [17]. Similarly, the pentagon task may lack accuracy in post-stroke, frontotemporal and subcortical dementias [18].

Low mood and depression may also impact on cognition and may precede onset of cognitive decline, affecting executive function, memory, and attention [19,20]. While evidence suggests that depression in MCI is associated with disease progression, the effects of depression on cognitive screening are poorly characterised [21]. Limited data suggests that mood may negatively influence MMSE scores, underestimating true performance [22]. The extent to which depression affects the results of the MMSE and other CSIs and their subtests is however, poorly understood and the extent to which different dementia subtype scores are influenced by the presence of comorbid depression is not known.

Although several studies have compared the diagnostic accuracy of the newer and shorter Q*mci* screen and shown it is better able to differentiate MCI from mild dementia and normal cognition than the SMMSE [8,13], to date, this has only been examined in those with Alzheimer's and vascular type dementia. The objective of this study is therefore to explore the performance (diagnostic accuracy) of these instruments across a broad range of different dementia subtypes, and in patients with MCI and those with and without depression. More broadly, this also serves to investigate the extent to which CSI's perform differently in these settings.

2. Methods

2.1. Data Collection

This study compared the SMMSE and the Q*mci* screen in patients (*n* = 3020) obtained from three geriatric and memory clinics in Canada over the decade between 1999 and 2010. Data were collected and analysed retrospectively from two clinic databases and a randomised controlled clinical trial dataset: The Geriatric Assessment Tool (GAT) [23], the Q*mci* screen original validation [8], and the Doxycycline and Rifampicin for Alzheimer's Disease (DARAD) Trial databases [24]. Recruitment processes from all three studies have been published previously [8,23,24]. In summary, the GAT is a customised software application that automates clinicians' outpatient reviews [23]. These data were collected in outpatient geriatric and memory clinics in two university hospitals in Ontario, Canada between 1999 and 2010. It contains approximately 8000 individual assessments from 1749 people aged 41–104 years. The Q*mci* screen validation database includes patients referred for assessment of cognition aged ≥55 years and recruited from four memory clinics in Ontario Canada [8]. The DARAD was a multi-centre, blinded, randomised trial conducted between 2006 and 2010, comparing the effect of rifampicin and doxycycline to placebo on the progression of AD [24]. The DARAD database includes patients ≥50 years with mild to moderate AD recruited from 14 centres across Canada. All three studies were led by the same principle investigator (D.W.M) and each participant underwent similar comprehensive work-up including laboratory investigations, neuropsychological assessment and neuroimaging where appropriate [23,24]. Ethical approval was obtained in advance for all three studies and participants provided informed written consent.

2.2. Participants

Participants were included in this analysis if both their SMMSE and Q*mci* screen scores were available. Participant selection is presented in Figure 1. MCI was diagnosed in patients presenting with subjective and objective memory loss, without loss of function. This was consistent with Petersen's criteria, where patients present with subjective memory complaints, objective abnormal memory function but preservation of activities of daily living and have no evidence of dementia [25]. Dementia was diagnosed using the Diagnostic and Statistical Manual of Mental Disorders (4th-edition) [26]. Mood was screened using the geriatric depression scale-short form with scores ≥5 assessed clinically for depression [27]. All participants were English literate. Those with MCI, predominantly amnestic type (aMCI), and patients with Alzheimer's disease (AD), vascular dementia (VaD), frontotemporal dementia (FTD), Lewy body dementia (LBD) and Parkinson's disease dementia (PDD), meeting established clinical criteria, with and without a history of comorbid depression, were included. Patients without cognitive impairment and with depression as the primary symptom were excluded. Persons attending with patients without memory loss (mainly caregivers) were recruited by convenience sampling as normal controls ($n = 875$).

2.3. Outcome Measures

The SMMSE is a standardised form of the MMSE developed to improve inter-rater reliability and reduced administration time by using explicit administration and scoring guidelines [2,3]. Scored out of 30 points, a score of 25/30 or more suggests that the individual may have normal cognition. Below this, scores can indicate mild (21–24 points), moderate (10–20 points) and severe cognitive impairment (≤9 points), though a cut-off of <24/30 optimises sensitivity [2,3]. It covers several cognitive domains including orientation, registration, delayed (verbal) recall, attention (concentration and calculation), language (including writing, reading and naming), command following, and visuospatial (construction) subtests [2,3]. The Q*mci* screen is a more recently developed short CSI, designed to separate MCI from mild dementia [8]. Scored from 100 points it incorporates six subtests across five cognitive domains including orientation, working memory, sematic memory (verbal fluency-categories), visuo-spatial (clock drawing) and two tests of episodic memory: Delayed recall and logical memory (immediate verbal recall of short a story) [28]. It has an optimal cut-off score for cognitive impairment of <62/100 [13,29]. It has been validated against the MoCA and different neuropsychological tests and is published in multiple languages [30–34]. While data on total scores were available for both CSIs, data on subtests were only available for the Q*mci* screen as these were not collected as part of the DARAD trial [24].

2.4. Analysis

Data were analysed using SPSS 24.0. Data from the three data sets (original Q*mci* screen validation database, GAT and DARAD datasets) were pooled and analysed using simple descriptive statistics. Data were non-normally distributed and were analysed with non-parametric tests. The Mann–Whitney U test was used to compare distributions between variables. Receiver operating characteristic (ROC) curve analysis was used to determine diagnostic accuracy from the area under the curve (AUC). AUC scores range from 0.5–1.0; 0.5 equates to chance alone and 1.0 perfect predictive accuracy. Scores from 0.50–0.59 indicate no or very poor accuracy, 0.60–0.69 poor, 0.70–0.79 fair, 0.80–0.89 good and 0.90–1.0 excellent to perfect accuracy [35]. All AUC values are presented with 95% confidence intervals (CI) and where specified were compared using the DeLong method [36]. Optimal cut-off points were calculated using Youden's Index.

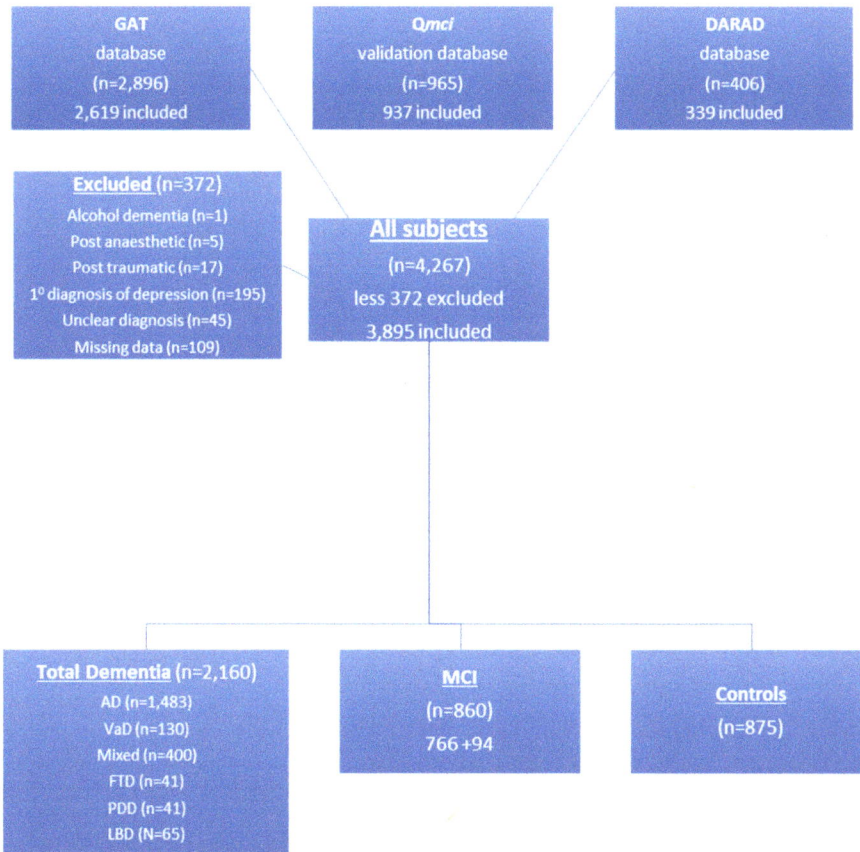

Figure 1. Flow chart presenting the recruitment of participants pooled from three data sets: The Geriatric Assessment Tool (GAT), Quick Mild Cognitive Impairment (Q*mci*) Screen and Doxycycline and Rifampicin for Alzheimer's Disease (DARAD) trial databases; it includes the number of controls, those with mild cognitive impairment (MCI) and specific dementia subtypes: Alzheimer's disease (AD), vascular dementia (VaD), mixed dementia, frontotemporal dementia (FTD), Parkinson's disease dementia (PDD) and Lewy body dementia (LBD) subtypes.

3. Results

In all, 3020 patients were available for analysis. A further 875 normal controls were included. The majority of participants had dementia (n = 2160) of which AD was the most common subtype (n = 1483), followed by mixed (AD-VaD) (n = 400) and VaD (n = 130). The median age of patients presenting with cognitive symptoms (MCI/dementia) was 77 years, interquartile range (IQR) ±9 compared to a median age of 69 (±14) years for normal controls, $p < 0.001$. In all, 51% of patients were male compared to 43% of controls, $p < 0.001$. Patients had completed a median of 12 (±5) years in education, similar to controls (13 ± 4), albeit statistically significantly lower, $p < 0.001$. The median SMMSE scores were 23/30 (±8) for dementia, 28/30 (±4) for MCI and 29/30 (±2) for controls. Median Q*mci* screen scores were 38/100 (±26) for dementia, 56/100 (±20) for MCI and 74/100 (±15) for controls. Differences in gender were seen between diagnosis with the percentage of males ranging from as high as 73% in those with VaD to as low as 41% in those with dementia and comorbid depression. Characteristics of participants including patients and controls are presented in Table 1.

Table 1. Characteristics of participants from the Quick Mild Cognitive Impairment (Qmci) Screen validation, Doxycycline And Rifampicin for Alzheimer's Disease study and Geriatric Assessment Tool databases, divided according to diagnosis: Depression, controls, mild cognitive impairment (MCI) and dementia including their Standardised Mini-Mental State Examination (SMMSE) and Qmci screen scores; comparison of SMMSE and Qmci screen score accuracy in differentiating each diagnosis from controls.

Diagnosis	N = X	Age (Median & IQR)	Education (Median & IQR)	Gender (% Male)	SMMSE (Median & IQR)	Qmci (Median & IQR)	SMMSE AUC NC v CI (95% Confidence Intervals)	Qmci AUC NC v CI (95% Confidence Intervals)	$p = x$
Total (All including co-morbid depression & MCI)	3020	77 (81 – 72 = 9)	12 (14 – 9 = 5)	1537/2997 * (51%)	25 (28 – 20 = 8)	43 (56 – 29 = 27)	0.87 (0.85–0.88)	0.93 (0.92–0.94)	$z = 11.6$ $p < 0.001$
Dementia (All including co-morbid depression)	2160	77 (82 – 73 = 9)	12 (14 – 9 = 5)	1087/2145 * (51%)	23 (26 – 18 = 8)	38 (50 – 24 = 26)	0.92 (0.91–0.93)	0.96 (0.95–0.96)	$z = -8.6$ $p < 0.001$
Dementia (All excluding co-morbid depression)	1879	78 (82 – 74 = 8)	11 (14 – 9 = 5)	971/1864 * (52%)	23 (26 – 18 = 8)	37 (49 – 24 = 25)	0.92 (0.91–0.93)	0.96 (0.95–0.97)	$z = -8.3$ $p < 0.001$
AD	1483	78 (83 – 74 = 9)	12 (14 – 9 = 5)	651/1475 * (44%)	23 (25.5 – 18 = 7.5)	37 (48 – 23 = 25)	0.94 (0.93–0.95)	0.97 (0.96–0.97)	$z = -5.9$ $p < 0.001$
VaD	130	74 (79 – 69 = 10)	12 (14 – 10 = 4)	95 (73%)	27 (29 – 25 = 4)	53 (64 – 40 = 24)	0.74 (0.68–0.79)	0.87 (0.84–0.91)	$z = -6.3$ $p < 0.001$
Mixed (AD/VaD)	400	77 (81 – 74 = 7)	11 (13 – 9 = 4)	256/393 * (65%)	22 (27 – 19 = 8)	36 (51 – 23 = 28)	0.91 (0.89–0.93)	0.95 (0.94–0.96)	$z = -5.7$ $p < 0.001$
AD, VaD and Mixed	2013	78 (82 – 74 = 4)	12 (14 – 9 = 5)	1002/1998 * (50%)	23 (26 – 18 = 8)	38 (50 – 24 = 26)	0.92 (0.91–0.93)	0.96 (0.95–0.97)	$z = 8.4$ $p < 0.001$
FTD	41	69 (71 – 62 = 9)	12 (14 – 10 = 4)	25/41 (61%)	23 (27 – 19 = 8)	42 (52 – 28 = 24)	0.90 (0.85–0.96)	0.96 (0.94–0.98)	$z = -2.5$ $p = 0.01$
PDD	41	75 (77 – 71 = 6)	12 (12 – 9.5 = 2.5)	28/41 (68%)	26 (29 – 21 = 8)	46 (61 – 32 = 29)	0.81 (0.72–0.90)	0.92 (0.88–0.95)	$z = -3.1$ $p = 0.002$
LBD	65	78 (82 – 73 = 9)	10 (14 – 8 = 6)	32/65 (49%)	24 (27 – 18 = 9)	37 (54 – 24 = 30)	0.94 (0.92–0.97)	0.94 (0.91–0.97)	$z = 0.11$ $p = 0.91$
MCI	860	75 (80 – 70 = 10)	12 (14 – 10 = 4)	450/852 * (53%)	28 (29 – 25 = 4)	56 (66 – 46 = 20)	0.73 (0.71–0.75)	0.85 (0.83–0.87)	$z = -10.8$ $p < 0.001$
Co-morbid depression	281	75 (81 – 70 = 11)	12 (14 – 10 = 4)	116/281 (41%)	25 (27 – 21 = 6)	44 (56 – 30 = 26)	0.88 (0.86–0.91)	0.93 (0.91–0.95)	$z = -4.2$ $p < 0.001$
MCI with co-morbid depression	94	73 (75 – 68 = 7)	12 (14 – 9 = 5)	50/92 * (54%)	26 (29 – 23 = 6)	52 (62 – 40 = 22)	0.79 (0.73–0.85)	0.90 (0.86–0.93)	$z = -4.4$ $p < 0.001$
MCI without co-morbid depression	766	76 (80 – 70 = 10)	12 (14 – 10 = 4)	400/760 * (53%)	28 (29 – 26 = 3)	57 (66 – 46 = 20)	0.72 (0.70–0.75)	0.84 (0.82–0.86)	$z = -10.4$ $p < 0.001$
Controls	875	70 (76 – 62 = 14)	13 (16 – 12 = 4)	372/875 (43%)	29 (30 – 28 = 2)	74 (81 – 66 = 15)	NA	NA	NA

AUC = area under the curve, AD = Alzheimer's disease, CI = cognitive impairment, FTD = frontotemporal dementia, IQR = interquartile range, LBD = Lewy body dementia, PDD = Parkinson's dementia, VaD = vascular dementia; NA = Not applicable;* Missing data.

Both instruments accurately differentiated cognitive impairment (MCI or dementia) from normal, although the Q*mci* screen was statistically more accurate than the SMMSE (AUC of 0.93 versus 0.87, respectively, *p* < 0.001). The SMMSE, at a cut-off of <24/30, had a sensitivity of 42%, specificity of 99% with a positive predictive value of 99% and negative predictive value of 33%. The Q*mci* screen had a sensitivity of 83% and specificity of 87% with a positive predictive value of 96% and negative predictive value of 60% at its published optimal cut-off score (<62/100). Using Youden's Index, the optimal cut-off scores for the SMMSE was 28/30, which gave a sensitivity of 75% and specificity of 88%. The optimal cut-off for the Q*mci* screen was <62. The SMMSE most accurately differentiated AD (AUC 0.94, 95% CI: 0.93–0.95) and LBD (AUC 0.94, 95% CI: 0.92–0.97) and least accurately identified MCI (AUC 0.73, 95% CI: 0.71–0.75), VaD (AUC 0.74, 95% CI: 0.68–0.79) and PDD (AUC 0.81, 95% CI: 0.72–0.90). The Q*mci* screen had statistically greater accuracy in distinguishing all dementia subtypes except LBD (*p* = 0.91). The Q*mci* screen was more accurate than the SMMSE in separating PDD and FTD from controls, albeit sample sizes were small. As expected, the Q*mci* screen had the greatest diagnostic accuracy for identifying MCI (AUC 0.85, 95% CI: 0.83-0.87) from normal controls, which was statistically significantly greater than the SMMSE (AUC 0.73, 95% CI: 0.71–0.75), *p* < 0.001. ROC curves demonstrating the accuracy of both instruments in each type of dementia, in MCI and in those with and without depression are presented in Figure 2a–l.

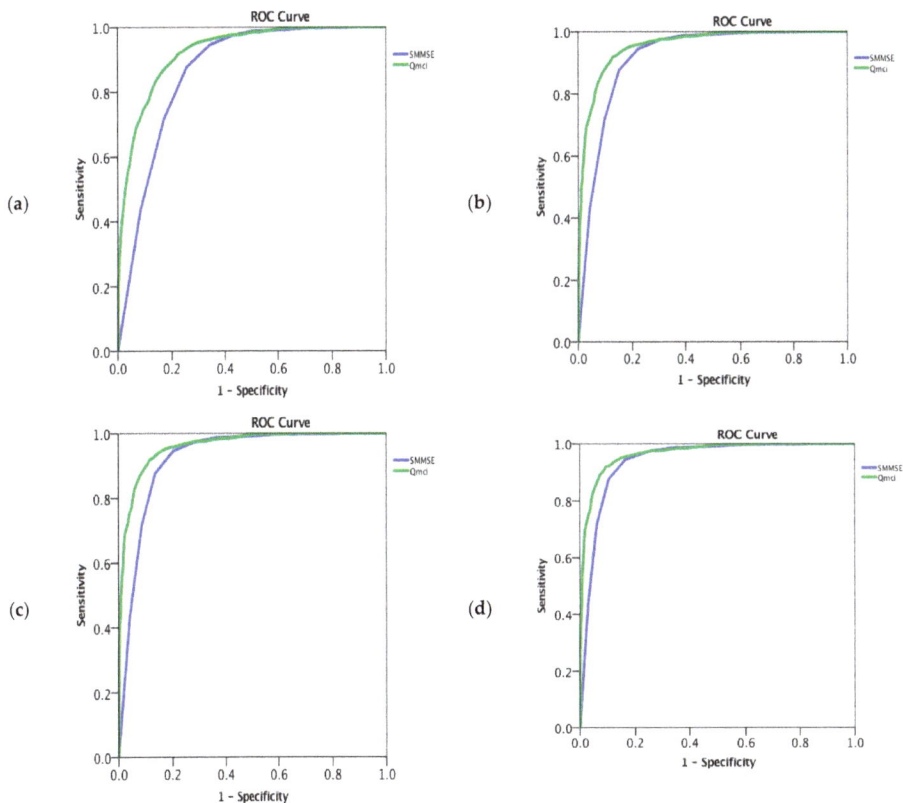

Figure 2. *Cont.*

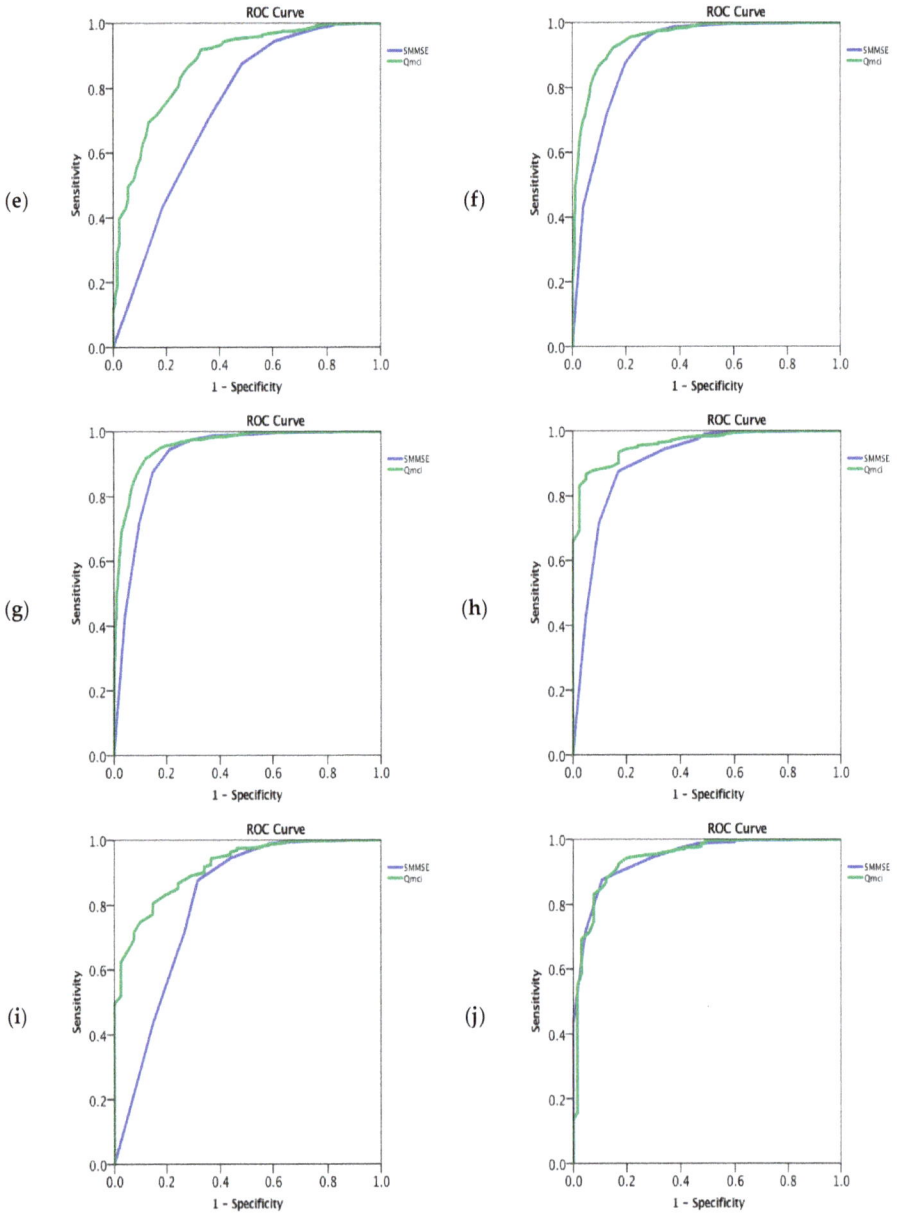

Figure 2. *Cont.*

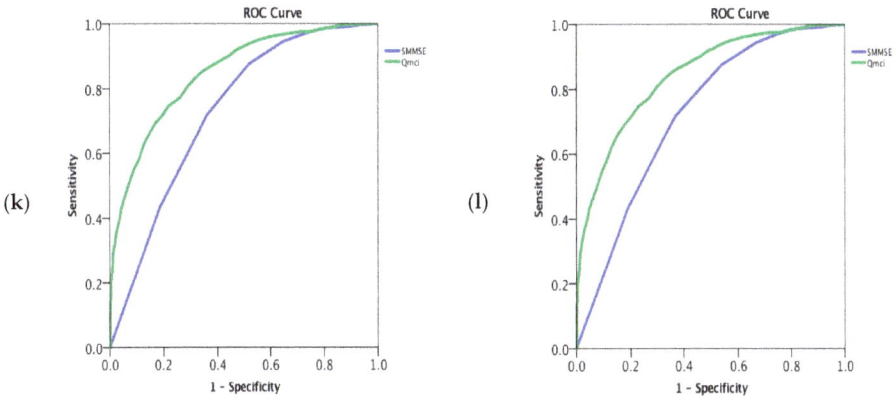

Figure 2. Receiver operating characteristic curves (**a–l**) comparing the accuracy of the Quick Mild Cognitive Impairment (Q*mci*) Screen and the Standardised Mini-Mental State Examination in differentiating normal controls (*n* = 875) from those with mild cognitive impairment (MCI), different dementia subtypes and comorbid depression for participants included within the Q*mci* screen validation, Doxycycline And Rifampicin for Alzheimer's Disease study and Geriatric Assessment Tool databases. (**a**). All patients (*n* = 3020); (**b**). All patients with dementia (*n* = 2160); (**c**). Dementia excluding depression (*n* = 1879); (**d**). Alzheimer's dementia (*n* = 1483); (**e**). Vascular dementia (*n* = 130); (**f**). Mixed dementia (*n* = 400); (**g**). Alzheimer's, vascular, mixed dementia (*n* = 2013); (**h**). Frontotemporal dementia (*n* = 41) (**i**). Parkinson's disease dementia (*n* = 41); (**j**). Lewy body dementia (*n* = 65); (**k**). All MCI (*n* = 860); (**l**) MCI excluding depression (*n* = 766).

The median subtest scores and AUC scores derived from ROC curves according to diagnosis are presented in Tables 2 and 3, respectively.

Table 2. Median scores for the Quick Mild Cognitive Impairment (*Qmci*) Screen subtests divided according to diagnosis: Depression, mild cognitive impairment (MCI) and dementia.

Diagnosis	N = X	Orientation (Median and IQR)	Registration (Median and IQR)	Clock Drawing (Median and IQR)	Delayed Recall (Median and IQR)	Verbal Fluency (Median and IQR)	Logical Memory (Median and IQR)	*Qmci* Total (Median and IQR)
Total (All)	3020	8 (10 – 6 = 4)	5 (5 – 4 = 1)	12 (14 – 5 = 9)	4 (12 – 0 = 12)	5 (7 – 3 = 4)	8 (12 – 4 = 8)	43 (56 – 29 = 27)
Dementia (All including co-morbid depression)	2160	7 (9 – 5 = 4)	5 (5 – 3 = 2)	11 (14 – 3 = 11)	4 (8 – 0 = 8)	5 (7 – 3 = 4)	8 (12 – 4 = 8)	38 (50 – 24 = 26)
Dementia (All excluding co-morbid depression)	1879	7 (9 – 5 = 4)	5 (5 – 3 = 2)	11 (13 – 3 = 10)	0 (8 – 0 = 8)	4 (6 – 3 = 3)	8 (12 – 4 = 8)	37 (49 – 24 = 25)
AD	1483	7 (9 – 5 = 4)	5 (5 – 3 = 2)	11 (13 – 3 = 10)	0 (8 – 0 = 8)	4 (6 – 3 = 3)	8 (12 – 4 = 8)	37 (48 – 23 = 25)
VaD	130	9 (10 – 7 = 3)	5 (5 – 4 = 1)	14 (15 – 11 = 4)	8 (12 – 0 = 12)	7 (9 – 4 = 5)	10 (14 – 8 = 6)	53 (64 – 40 = 24)
Mixed (AD/VaD)	400	7 (10 – 5 = 5)	5 (5 – 3 = 2)	10 (14 – 2 = 12)	0 (8 – 0 = 8)	5 (7 – 3 = 4)	8 (12 – 4 = 8)	35.5 (51 – 23 = 28)
AD, VaD and Mixed	2013	7 (9 – 5 = 4)	5 (5 – 3 = 2)	11 (14 – 3 = 11)	0 (8 – 0 = 8)	5 (7 – 3 = 4)	8 (12 – 4 = 8)	38 (50 – 24 = 26)
FTD	41	9 (10 – 6 = 4)	5 (5 – 3 = 2)	12 (13 – 5 = 8)	4 (8 – 0 = 8)	4 (7 – 3 = 4)	8 (12 – 4 = 8)	43 (55 – 30 = 25)
PDD	41	9.5 (10 – 7 = 3)	5 (5 – 4 = 1)	12.5 (15 – 7 = 8)	8 (12 – 0 = 12)	5.5 (7 – 4 = 3)	10 (14 – 8 = 6)	46 (61 – 32 = 29)
LBD	65	8 (10 – 6 = 4)	5 (5 – 3 = 2)	7 (12 – 1 = 11)	8 (12 – 0 = 12)	4 (6 – 3 = 3)	8 (10 – 4 = 6)	37 (54 – 24 = 30)
MCI	860	10 (10 – 8 = 2)	5 (5 – 5 = 0)	14 (15 – 12 = 3)	12 (16 – 4 = 12)	7 (9 – 5 = 4)	12 (16 – 8 = 8)	56 (66 – 46 = 20)
Co-morbid depression	281	8 (10 – 6 = 4)	5 (5 – 4 = 1)	11 (14 – 4 = 10)	4 (12 – 0 = 12)	6 (8 – 3 = 5)	10 (14 – 4 = 10)	44 (56 – 30 = 26)
MCI with co-morbid depression	94	9 (10 – 7 = 3)	5 (5 – 4 = 1)	13 (15 – 10 = 5)	8 (12 – 4 = 8)	8 (8 – 4 = 4)	12 (14 – 8 = 6)	51.5 (62 – 40 = 22)
MCI without co-morbid depression	766	10 (10 – 8 = 2)	5 (5 – 5 = 0)	14 (15 – 12 = 3)	12 (16 – 4 = 12)	7 (9 – 5 = 4)	12 (16 – 8 = 8)	57 (66 – 46 = 20)
Controls	875	10 (10 – 10 = 0)	5 (5 – 5 = 0)	15 (15 – 14 = 1)	16 (20 – 12 = 8)	10 (13 – 8 = 5)	18 (22 – 14 = 8)	74 (81 – 66 = 15)

AD = Alzheimer's disease, FTD = frontotemporal dementia, LBD = Lewy body dementia, PDD = Parkinson's dementia, VaD = vascular dementia (IQR = interquartile range).

Table 3. Comparison of the accuracy of the Quick Mild Cognitive Impairment ($Qmci$) Screen subtests in differentiating each diagnosis from controls ($n = 875$): Depression, mild cognitive impairment (MCI) and dementia.

Diagnosis	$N = X$	Orientation AUC (95% CI)	Registration AUC (95% CI)	Clock Drawing AUC (95% CI)	Delayed Recall AUC (95% CI)	Verbal Fluency AUC (95% CI)	Logical Memory AUC (95% CI)	$Qmci$ Total AUC (95% CI)
Total (All)	3020	0.81 (0.79–0.82)	0.62 (0.60–0.64)	0.80 (0.79–0.82)	0.86 (0.85–0.87)	0.85 (0.84–0.87)	0.87 (0.85–0.88)	0.93 (0.92–0.94)
Dementia (All including co-morbid depression)	2160	0.86 (0.85–0.87)	0.65 (0.63–0.67)	0.85 (0.83–0.86)	0.90 (0.89–0.91)	0.89 (0.88–0.90)	0.89 (0.88–0.91)	0.96 (0.95–0.96)
Dementia (All excluding co-morbid depression)	1879	0.87 (0.85–0.88)	0.66 (0.64–0.68)	0.85 (0.84–0.87)	0.90 (0.89–0.92)	0.90 (0.88–0.91)	0.90 (0.89–0.91)	0.96 (0.95–0.97)
AD	1483	0.88 (0.87–0.90)	0.66 (0.64–0.68)	0.85 (0.84–0.87)	0.91 (0.90–0.93)	0.91 (0.89–0.92)	0.91 (0.89–0.92)	0.97 (0.96–0.97)
VaD	130	0.71 (0.66–0.77)	0.56 (0.50–0.61)	0.72 (0.67–0.77)	0.80 (0.75–0.84)	0.80 (0.77–0.84)	0.81 (0.77–0.85)	0.87 (0.84–0.91)
Mixed (AD/VaD)	400	0.84 (0.82–0.87)	0.65 (0.61–0.68)	0.85 (0.82–0.87)	0.90 (0.88–0.92)	0.89 (0.87–0.91)	0.89 (0.87–0.91)	0.95 (0.94–0.96)
AD, VaD & Mixed	2013	0.86 (0.85–0.88)	0.65 (0.63–0.67)	0.84 (0.83–0.86)	0.90 (0.89–0.91)	0.90 (0.88–0.91)	0.90 (0.88–0.91)	0.96 (0.95–0.97)
FTD	41	0.78 (0.69–0.87)	0.63 (0.53–0.73)	0.88 (0.81–0.94)	0.90 (0.87–0.95)	0.85 (0.78–0.92)	0.88 (0.83–0.93)	0.96 (0.94–0.98)
PDD	41	0.71 (0.61–0.81)	0.68 (0.58–0.77)	0.73 (0.63–0.82)	0.84 (0.77–0.91)	0.85 (0.79–0.91)	0.83 (0.77–0.88)	0.92 (0.88–0.95)
LBD	65	0.82 (0.74–0.88)	0.66 (0.58–0.74)	0.92 (0.87–0.96)	0.84 (0.79–0.90)	0.89 (0.85–0.93)	0.86 (0.81–0.92)	0.94 (0.91–0.97)
MCI	860	0.68 (0.65–0.70)	0.54 (0.51–0.57)	0.69 (0.67–0.72)	0.76 (0.74–0.78)	0.76 (0.74–0.78)	0.80 (0.77–0.81)	0.85 (0.83–0.87)
Co-morbid depression	281	0.80 (0.77–0.84)	0.62 (0.57–0.66)	0.81 (0.78–0.84)	0.86 (0.84–0.89)	0.84 (0.82–0.87)	0.84 (0.82–0.87)	0.93 (0.91–0.95)
MCI with co-morbid depression	94	0.75 (0.69–0.82)	0.59 (0.52–0.65)	0.75 (0.70–0.81)	0.82 (0.78–0.87)	0.80 (0.76–0.85)	0.80 (0.75–0.84)	0.90 (0.86–0.93)
MCI without co-morbid depression	766	0.67 (0.64–0.69)	0.53 (0.50–0.56)	0.69 (0.66–0.71)	0.75 (0.73–0.77)	0.76 (0.73–0.78)	0.80 (0.76–0.81)	0.84 (0.82–0.86)

AD = Alzheimer's disease, FTD = frontotemporal dementia, LBD = Lewy body dementia, PDD = Parkinson's dementia, VaD = vascular dementia; AUC = area under the curve; CI = confidence intervals.

ROC curves comparing the subtests of the Q*mci* screen are presented in Figure 3a–l. The highest median score for the clock drawing subtest was found in those with VaD (14/15), the lowest was in LBD (7/15). The logical memory subtest was the most accurate of the Q*mci* screen subtests for most dementia subtypes and MCI (AUC 0.80, 95% CI: 0.77–0.81). Orientation was accurate for AD (AUC 0.88, 95% CI:) but had particularly low accuracy in VaD (AUC 0.71, 95% CI: 0.66–0.71), FTD (AUC 0.78, 95% CI: 0.69–0.87), PDD (AUC 0.71, 95% CI: 0.61–0.81) and MCI (AUC 0.68, 95% CI: 0.65–0.70). Clock drawing had the highest accuracy for identifying PDD (AUC 0.92, 95% CI: 0.87–0.96). Word registration had the lowest accuracy for all dementia subtypes and MCI.

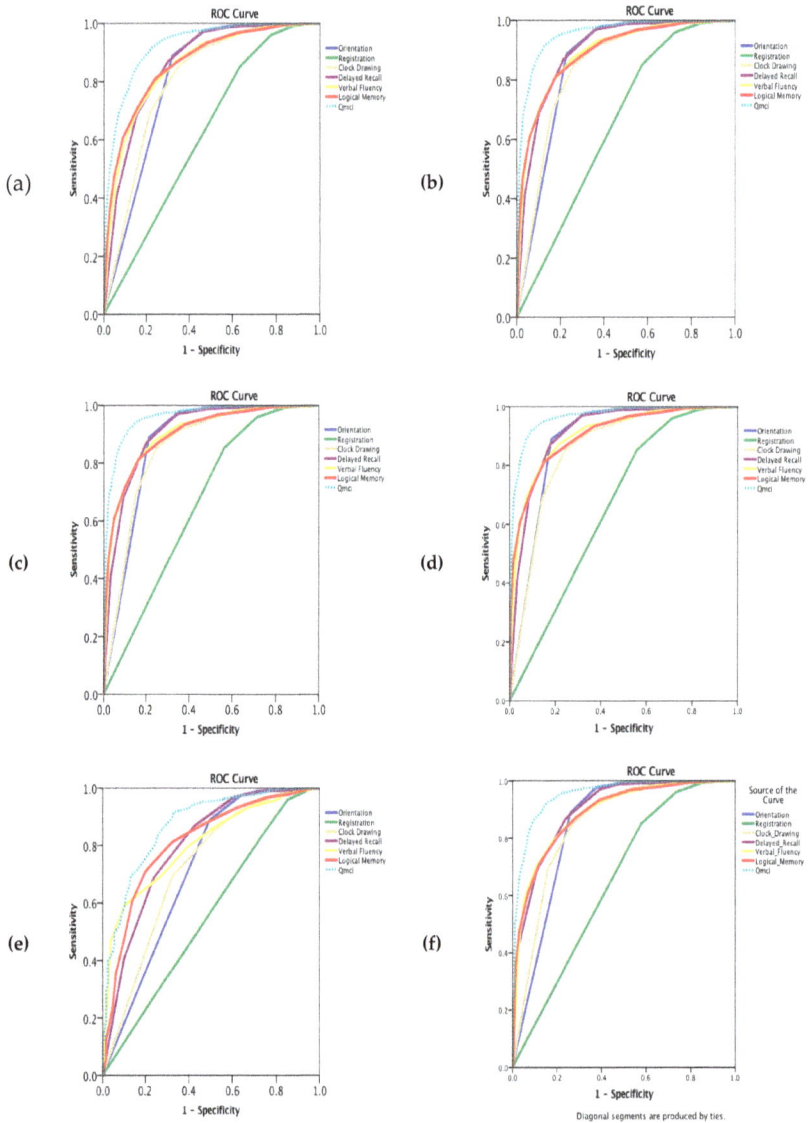

Figure 3. *Cont.*

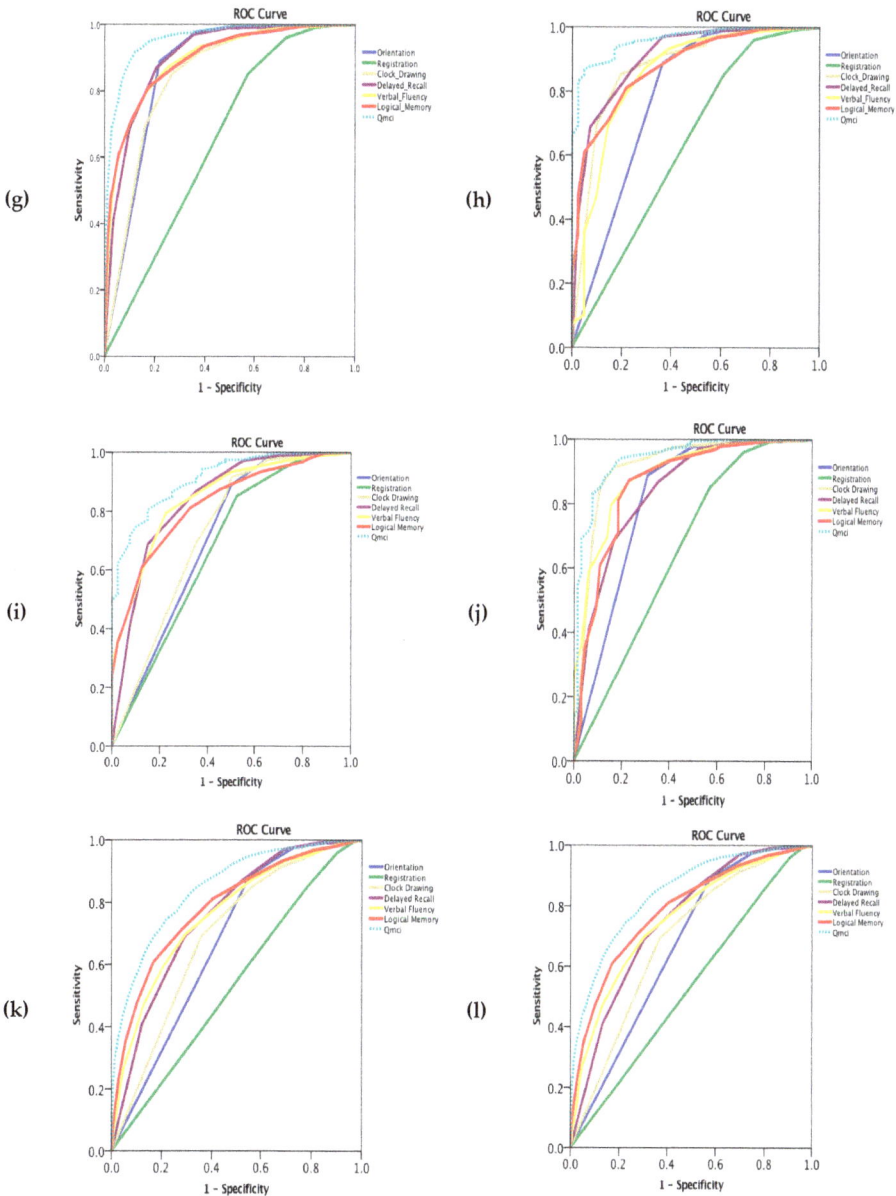

Figure 3. Receiver operating characteristic curves (**a–l**) comparing the accuracy of the Quick Mild Cognitive Impairment (Q*mci*) subtests in differentiating normal controls (*n* = 875) from those with mild cognitive impairment (MCI), different dementia subtypes and comorbid depression for participants included within the Q*mci* screen validation, Doxycycline and Rifampicin for Alzheimer's Disease study and Geriatric Assessment Tool databases. (**a**). All patients (*n* = 3020); (**b**). All patients with dementia (*n* = 2160); (**c**). Dementia excluding depression (*n* = 1879); (**d**). Alzheimer's dementia (*n* = 1483); (**e**). Vascular dementia (*n* = 130); (**f**). Mixed dementia (*n* = 400); (**g**). Alzheimer's, vascular, mixed dementia (*n* = 2013); (**h**). Frontotemporal dementia (*n* = 41); (**i**). Parkinson's disease dementia (*n* = 41); (**j**). Lewy body dementia (*n* = 65); (**k**). All MCI (*n* = 860); (**l**). MCI excluding depression (*n* = 766).

Diagnostics **2019**, *9*, 93

Those diagnosed with dementia and co-morbid depression were younger ($z = -5.9$, $p < 0.001$) and more likely to be female ($X^2 = 11.4$, $p < 0.001$) than those without comorbid depression. There was no statistically significant difference in the number of years in education ($z = -1.3$, $p = 0.21$). Those diagnosed with dementia (all subtypes excluding MCI) with co-morbid depression ($n = 281$) had statistically significantly higher median Q*mci* screen and SMMSE scores than those without ($n = 1879$) depression: Median Q*mci* screen scores of 44 versus 37, respectively ($z = -4.771$, $p < 0.001$) and median SMMSE scores of 25 versus 23, respectively ($z = -5.627$, $p < 0.001$). Contrasting this, comparison of median scores for MCI with and without depression showed that scores were significantly lower for those with co-morbid depression for both the Q*mci* screen, (52 and 57 respectively, $z = -2.927$, $p = 0.003$) and SMMSE (26 and 28 respectively, $z = -3.302$, $p = 0.001$). Co-morbid depression lowered the diagnostic accuracy of both instruments for dementia but improved the accuracy in those with MCI. All Q*mci* screen subtest scores were less accurate for MCI among those patients with co-morbid depression.

4. Discussion

This study compares the diagnostic accuracy of the SMMSE and Q*mci* screen in different dementia subtypes using a large sample of patients pooled from three different datasets using AUC values as a global measure of diagnostic accuracy. The results show that the SMMSE and Q*mci* screen are both accurate CSIs when used to identify dementia in patients presenting with cognitive symptoms to geriatric and memory clinics compared with normal controls. Overall, the Q*mci* screen had high sensitivity and specificity in separating normal controls from those with cognitive impairment (MCI or dementia with or with co-morbid depression). The SMMSE had poor sensitivity, albeit excellent specificity at its widely-used cut-off. These results would be expected as the Q*mci* screen contains more challenging tests of episodic memory [28], which are better able to differentiate MCI from mild dementia [8,29]. The SMMSE is overly weighted towards tests of orientation (one-third of its points), which is best able to identify established dementia [28]. Further, while a cut-off of <24/30 is widely applied for the SMMSE, recent studies suggest that higher cut-offs between 26 [37] and 29 [13], closer to that found here, are more accurate and produce a better balance between sensitivity and specificity. As with its' original validation study [8,28], this analysis confirms the Q*mci* screen is more accurate overall and that its logical memory subtest is its most accurate for separating MCI from normal controls. It also had high levels of accuracy for most dementia subtypes and patients with and without co-morbid depression. The SMMSE, while it had good to excellent accuracy in differentiating most dementia subtypes from normal controls, was less accurate in identifying MCI [8], and had only fair accuracy in identifying VaD (AUC of 0.74) from controls, supporting previous studies in these conditions, where an alternative instrument is suggested [17]. Similarly, while the SMMSE's accuracy in detecting PDD from normal controls was good (AUC 0.81), it performed relatively poorly compared to the Q*mci* screen, supporting evidence that it is less suitable due to both floor and ceiling effects in those with movement disorders [18,38]. The study also examined the subtests of the Q*mci* screen and their differential accuracy in separating those with MCI and dementia from normal controls. As was found in the initial validation, logical memory was most accurate in identifying MCI [28]. Clock drawing was most accurate in detecting LBD but the accuracy for PDD was relatively lower. Clock drawing is often grossly abnormal in LBD, particularly for copying rather than drawing clocks [39]. Differences between LBD and PDD were unexpected and it is likely that small numbers influenced the results. Orientation was only accurate for AD and mixed dementia having poor accuracy for other dementia subtypes and MCI.

In this study, co-morbid depression had a significant impact on CSI scores; those with dementia and depression scored significantly higher on both the SMMSE and Q*mci* screen than those without. This was unexpected as other studies [22] suggest that impaired attention and other cognitive deficits associated with low mood negatively impact on scores. Nevertheless, co-morbid depression did lower the diagnostic accuracy of both instruments for differentiating dementia from normal controls.

The opposite effect was seen for MCI; those with co-morbid depression scored less well on both CSIs, which had higher diagnostic accuracy for these patients. This suggests that comorbid depression may influence CSIs in different ways depending on the diagnostic stage of cognitive impairment. Depression may also have a greater clinical effect at earlier stages of disease progression with evidence that depressive symptoms increase the risk for converting from MCI to dementia, particularly amnestic type to AD [21,40].

The strength of this study is derived from its large sample size and careful pooling of data derived from similar data sets collected by the same principal investigator. This study also has limitations. Pooling data from discrete, albeit related, datasets with different populations may have created bias. Some data on gender were missing and subtest data for the SMMSE were not available across all three datasets, which limited the analysis. The number of patients with atypical or less common dementia subtypes was small and may be unrepresentative of the true performance of the instruments in that subtype, leading to bias. The data collection began in 1999 when the awareness of LBD was low, potentially resulting in misclassification bias. Likewise, only patients with AD or those with AD, VaD and mixed dementia were included in the DARAD and the Q*mci* validation databases respectively. In addition, the prevalence of cognitive impairment (MCI/dementia) was high among those attending these geriatric and memory clinics potentially leading to spectrum bias. Further, this study was a retrospective review of patients with no detailed information available regarding the type of depressive symptoms. Similarly, it was not possible to assess MCI subtypes in this study, though the majority of patients in the GAT database reported amnestic type symptoms, suggesting that most had aMCI. Finally, the statistical analysis was limited to using AUC scores as a global measure of diagnostic accuracy and further research is now planned to explore the psychometric properties of these instruments in different dementia subtypes and to identify the optimal cut-off scores.

In summary, this study reaffirms that both the SMMSE and Q*mci* screen are useful in separating patients with dementia from normal controls. It confirms the superior accuracy of the Q*mci* screen in MCI. It also shows that different short screens have significantly different accuracy in different dementia subtypes, suggesting that pre-screen/pre-test suspicion of a possible diagnosis (MCI or specific dementia subtype) based upon history and examination should direct the choice of instrument to be used when performing cognitive screening. This is important as time is limited in clinical practice and short CSIs can only include a limited number of domains, resulting in a time-accuracy trade-off supporting the need for careful selection a priori [41]. The results also suggest that a history of depression may affect the accuracy of cognitive screens, particularly in those with MCI in which it lowers median scores but increased the diagnostic accuracy of CSIs. The opposite effect was seen in dementia. This shows the importance of asking about depression when undertaking cognitive screening [20] and that the effect of comorbid depression on cognitive screening scores merits further investigation. Understanding the optimal cut-offs for these instruments and other short CSIs is also important, so that not only the most appropriate instrument is used in the right setting but also the correct cut-off score is applied. To date, no condition-specific cut-off scores for the SMMSE or Q*mci* screen are available, highlighting that this is an area requiring more research. Further study is also required to confirm these findings and compare with sensitive and specific instruments such as the MoCA and the Mini-Addenbrooke's Cognitive Examination [42].

Author Contributions: R.O. and D.W.M. conceived and designed the study; D.W.M. collected the data; R.O. analyzed the data; R.O. wrote the initial draft of the paper. R.O. and D.W.M. reviewed the submitted and revised drafts.

Funding: This research received no external funding.

Acknowledgments: Yang Gao for his role in data preparation and analysis of these datasets.

Conflicts of Interest: R.O. and D.W.M. are co-copyright holders of the Quick Mild Cognitive Impairment (Q*mci*) screen; D.W.M. is the sole copyright holder of the Standardised Mini-Mental State Examination. The authors declare no other conflicts of interest.

References

1. Folstein, M.F.; Folstein, S.E.; McHugh, P.R. "Mini-Mental State". A practical method for grading the cognitive state of patients for the clinician. *J. Psychiatry Res.* **1975**, *12*, 189–198. [CrossRef]
2. Molloy, D.W.; Alemayehu, E.; Roberts, R. Reliability of a Standardized Mini-Mental State Examination compared with the traditional Mini-Mental State Examination. *Am. J. Psychiatry* **1991**, *148*, 102–105. [CrossRef] [PubMed]
3. Molloy, D.W.; Standish, T.I.M. A guide to the Standardized Mini-Mental State Examination. *Int. Psychogeriatry* **1997**, *9*, 87–94. [CrossRef]
4. Woodford, H.J.; George, J. Cognitive assessment in the elderly: A review of clinical methods. *QJM Int. J. Med.* **2007**, *100*, 469–484. [CrossRef] [PubMed]
5. Breton, A.; Casey, D.; Arnaoutoglou, N.A. Cognitive tests for the detection of mild cognitive impairment (MCI), the prodromal stage of dementia: Meta-analysis of diagnostic accuracy studies. *Int. J. Geriatr. Psychiatry* **2019**, *34*, 233–242. [CrossRef] [PubMed]
6. Albert, M.S.; DeKosky, S.T.; Dickson, D.; Dubois, B.; Feldman, H.H.; Fox, N.C.; Snyder, P.J. The diagnosis of mild cognitive impairment due to Alzheimer's disease: Recommendations from the national institute on aging-Alzheimer's association workgroups on diagnostic guidelines for Alzheimer's disease. *Alzheimers Dement.* **2011**, *7*, 270–279. [CrossRef]
7. Rami, L.; Molinuevo, J.L.; Sanchez-Valle, R.; Bosch, B.; Villar, A. Screening for amnestic mild cognitive impairment and early Alzheimer's disease with M@T (Memory Alteration Test) in the primary care population. *Int. J. Geriatr. Psychiatry* **2007**, *22*, 294–304. [CrossRef]
8. O'Caoimh, R.; Gao, Y.; McGlade, C.; Healy, L.; Gallagher, P.; Timmons, S.; Molloy, D.W. Comparison of the Quick Mild Cognitive Impairment (Qmci) screen and the SMMSE in screening for mild cognitive impairment. *Age Ageing* **2012**, *41*, 624–629. [CrossRef]
9. Nasreddine, Z.S.; Phillips, N.A.; Bédirian, V.; Charbonneau, S.; Whitehead, V.; Collin, I.; Cummings, J.L.; Chertkow, H. The Montreal Cognitive Assessment, MoCA: A brief screening tool for mild cognitive impairment. *J. Am. Geriatr. Soc.* **2005**, *53*, 695–699. [CrossRef]
10. Mitchell, A.J. A Meta-Analysis of the Accuracy of the Mini-Mental State Examination in the Detection of Dementia and Mild Cognitive Impairment. *J. Psychiatry Res.* **2009**, *43*, 411–431. [CrossRef]
11. Mitchell, A.J.; Shiri-Feshki, M. Rate of progression of mild cognitive impairment to dementia-meta-analysis of 41 robust inception cohort studies. *Acta Psychiatry Scand.* **2009**, *119*, 252–265. [CrossRef] [PubMed]
12. Crum, R.M.; Anthony, J.C.; Bassett, S.S.; Folstein, M.F. Population-based norms for the Mini-Mental State Examination by age and educational level. *J. Am. Med. Assoc.* **1993**, *269*, 2386–2391. [CrossRef]
13. O'Caoimh, R.; Gao, Y.; Svendovski, A.; Gallagher, P.; Eustace, J.; Molloy, D.W. Comparing approaches to optimize cut-off scores for short cognitive screening instruments in mild cognitive impairment and dementia. *J. Alzheimers Dis.* **2017**, *57*, 123–133. [CrossRef] [PubMed]
14. Velayudhan, L.; Ryu, S.H.; Raczek, M.; Philpot, M.; Lindesay, J.; Critchfield, M.; Livingston, G. Review of brief cognitive tests for patients with suspected dementia. *Int. Psychogeriatry* **2014**, *26*, 1247–1262. [CrossRef] [PubMed]
15. Nazem, S.; Siderowf, A.D.; Duda, J.E.; Have, T.T.; Colcher, A.; Horn, S.S.; Moberg, P.J.; Wilkinson, J.R.; Hurtig, H.I.; Stern, M.B.; et al. Montreal Cognitive Assessment performance in patients with Parkinson's disease with "normal" global cognition according to mini-mental state examination score. *J. Am. Geriatr. Soc.* **2009**, *57*, 304–308. [CrossRef] [PubMed]
16. Osher, J.E.; Wicklund, A.H.; Rademaker, A.; Johnson, N.; Weintraub, S. The Mini-Mental State Examination in behavioral variant frontotemporal dementia and primary progressive aphasia. *Am. J. Alzheimer's Dis.* **2008**, *22*, 468–473. [CrossRef] [PubMed]
17. Ghafar, M.Z.A.A.; Miptah, H.N.; O'Caoimh, R. Cognitive screening instruments to identify vascular cognitive impairment: A systematic review. *Int. J. Geriatr. Psychiatry* **2019**, *34*, 1114–1127. [CrossRef]
18. Bak, T.H.; Rogers, T.T.; Crawford, L.M.; Hearn, V.C.; Mathuranath, P.S.; Hodges, J.R. Cognitive bedside assessment in atypical parkinsonian syndromes. *J. Neurol. Neurosurg. Psychiatry* **2005**, *76*, 420–422. [CrossRef]
19. Russo, M.; Mahon, K.; Burdick, K. Measuring cognitive functions in MDD: Emerging assessment tools. *Depress. Anxiety* **2015**, *32*, 262–269. [CrossRef]

20. Richardson, L.; Adams, S. Cognitive deficits in patients with depression. *J. Nur. Pract.* **2018**, *14*, 437–443. [CrossRef]

21. Van der Mussele, S.; Fransen, E.; Struyfs, H.; Luyckx, J.; Mariën, P.; Saerens, J.; Somers, N.; Goeman, J.; De Deyn, P.P.; Engelborghs, S. Depression in Mild Cognitive Impairment is associated with Progression to Alzheimer's Disease: A Longitudinal Study. *J. Alzheimers Dis.* **2014**, *42*, 1239–1250. [CrossRef] [PubMed]

22. Anderson, T.M.; Sachdev, P.S.; Brodaty, H.; Trollor, J.N.; Andrews, G. Effects of sociodemographic and health variables on Mini-Mental State Exam scores in older Australians. *Am. J. Ger. Psychiatry* **2007**, *15*, 467–476. [CrossRef] [PubMed]

23. Gao, Y.; O'Caoimh, R.; Healy, L.; Kerins, D.M.; Eustace, J.; Guyatt, G.; Sammon, D.; Molloy, D.W. Effects of centrally acting ACE inhibitors on the rate of cognitive decline in dementia. *BMJ Open* **2013**, *3*, e002881. [CrossRef] [PubMed]

24. Molloy, D.W.; Standish, T.I.; Zhou, Q.; Guyatt, G. DARAD Study Group. A multicenter, blinded, randomized, factorial controlled trial of doxycycline and rifampin for treatment of Alzheimer's disease: The DARAD trial. *Int. J. Geriatr. Psychiatry* **2013**, *28*, 463–470. [CrossRef] [PubMed]

25. Petersen, R.C.; Smith, G.E.; Waring, S.C.; Ivnik, R.J.; Tangalos, E.G.; Kokmen, E. Mild cognitive impairment: Clinical characterization an outcome. *Arch. Neurol.* **1999**, *56*, 303–308. [CrossRef]

26. American Psychiatric Association. *Diagnostic and Statistical Manual of Mental Disorders*, 4th ed.; American Psychiatric Association: Washington, DC, USA, 1994.

27. Yesavage, J.A. Geriatric Depression Scale. *Psychopharmacol. Bull.* **1988**, *24*, 709–711.

28. O'Caoimh, R.; Gao, Y.; Gallagher, P.F.; Eustace, J.; McGlade, C.; Molloy, D.W. Which part of the Quick Mild Cognitive Impairment screen (Qmci) discriminates between normal cognition, mild cognitive impairment and dementia? *Age Ageing* **2013**, *42*, 324–330. [CrossRef]

29. O'Caoimh, R.; Timmons, S.; Molloy, D.W. Screening for Mild Cognitive Impairment: Comparison of "MCI Specific" Screening Instruments. *J. Alzheimer's Dis.* **2016**, *51*, 619–629. [CrossRef]

30. O'Caoimh, R.; Svendrovski, A.; Johnston, B.C.; Gao, Y.; McGlade, C.; Eustace, J.; Timmons, S.; Guyatt, G.; Molloy, D.W. The Quick Mild Cognitive Impairment screen correlated with the Standardized Alzheimer's Disease Assessment Scale–cognitive section in clinical trials. *J. Clin. Epidemiol.* **2014**, *67*, 87–92. [CrossRef]

31. Bunt, S.; O'Caoimh, R.; Krijnen, W.P.; Molloy, D.W.; Goodijk, G.P.; Van der Schans, C.P.; Hobbelen, H.J.S.M. Validation of the Dutch version of the quick mild cognitive impairment screen (Qmci-D). *BMC Geriatr.* **2015**, *15*, 115. [CrossRef]

32. Yavuz, B.B.; Varan, H.D.; O'Caoimh, R.; Kizilarslanoglu, M.C.; Kilic, M.K.; Molloy, D.W.; Dogrul, R.T.; Karabulut, E.; Svendrovski, A.; Sagir, A.; et al. Validation of the Turkish Version of the Quick Mild Cognitive Impairment Screen. *Am. J. Alzheimer's Dis.* **2017**, *32*, 145–156. [CrossRef] [PubMed]

33. Iavarone, A.; Carpinelli Mazzi, M.; Russo, G.; D'Anna, F.; Peluso, S.; Mazzeo, P.; De Luca, V.; De Michele, G.; Iaccarino, G.; Abete, P.; et al. The Italian version of the Quick Mild Cognitive Impairment (Qmci-I) screen: Normative study on 307 healthy subjects. *Aging Clin. Exp. Res.* **2018**, *31*, 353–360. [CrossRef] [PubMed]

34. Morita, A.; O'Caoimh, R.; Murayama, H.; Molloy, D.W.; Inoue, S.; Shobugawa, Y.; Fujiwara, T. Validity of the Japanese Version of the Quick Mild Cognitive Impairment Screen. *Int. J. Environ. Res. Public Health* **2019**, *16*, 917. [CrossRef] [PubMed]

35. Metz, C.E. Basic principles of ROC curve analysis. *Sem. Nucl. Med.* **1979**, *8*, 283–298. [CrossRef]

36. DeLong, E.R.; DeLong, D.M.; Clarke-Pearson, D.L. Comparing the areas under two or more correlated receiver operating characteristic curves: A nonparametric approach. *Biometrics* **1988**, *44*, 837–845. [CrossRef] [PubMed]

37. Kvitting, A.S.; Fällman, K.; Wressle, E.; Marcusson, J. Age-Normative MMSE Data for Older Persons Aged 85 to 93 in a Longitudinal Swedish Cohort. *J. Am. Geriatr. Soc.* **2019**, *67*, 534–538. [CrossRef] [PubMed]

38. Biundo, R.; Weis, L.; Bostantjopoulou, S.; Stefanova, E.; Falup-Pecurariu, C.; Kramberger, M.G.; Geurtsen, G.J.; Antonini, A.; Weintraub, D.; Aarsland, D. MMSE and MoCA in Parkinson's disease and dementia with Lewy bodies: A multicenter 1-year follow-up study. *J. Neural Transm.* **2016**, *123*, 431–438. [CrossRef] [PubMed]

39. Gnanalingham, K.K.; Byrne, E.J.; Thornton, A.; Sambrook, M.A.; Bannister, P. Motor and cognitive function in Lewy body dementia: Comparison with Alzheimer's and Parkinson's diseases. *J. Neur. Neurosurg. Psychiatry* **1997**, *62*, 243–252. [CrossRef] [PubMed]

40. Kida, J.; Nemoto, K.; Ikejima, C.; Bun, S.; Kakuma, T.; Mizukami, K.; Asada, T. Impact of depressive symptoms on conversion from mild cognitive impairment subtypes to Alzheimer's disease: A community-based longitudinal study. *J. Alzheimer's Dis.* **2016**, *51*, 405–415. [CrossRef] [PubMed]

41. Larner, A.J. MACE versus MoCA: Equivalence or superiority? Pragmatic diagnostic test accuracy study. *Int. Psychogeriatr.* **2017**, *29*, 931–937. [CrossRef] [PubMed]

42. Larner, A.J. Speed versus accuracy in cognitive assessment when using CSIs. *Prog. Neurol. Psychiatry* **2015**, *19*, 21–24. [CrossRef]

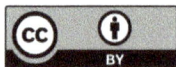

diagnostics

MDPI

Article

The Newly Normed SKT Reveals Differences in Neuropsychological Profiles of Patients with MCI, Mild Dementia and Depression

Hartmut Lehfeld [1,*] and Mark Stemmler [2]

[1] Department of Psychiatry and Psychotherapy, Paracelsus Medical University, 90419 Nuremberg, Germany
[2] Institute of Psychology, University of Erlangen-Nuremberg, 91052 Erlangen, Germany;
    mark.stemmler@fau.de
* Correspondence: Hartmut.Lehfeld@klinikum-nuernberg.de

Received: 18 July 2019; Accepted: 22 October 2019; Published: 25 October 2019

Abstract: The SKT (Syndrom-Kurztest) is a short cognitive performance test assessing deficits of memory and attention in the sense of speed of information processing. The new standardization of the SKT (2015) aimed at improving its sensitivity for early cognitive decline due to dementia in subjects aged 60 or older. The goal of this article is to demonstrate how the neuropsychological test profile of the SKT can be used to provide valuable information for a differential diagnosis between MCI (mild cognitive impairment), dementia and depression. $n = 549$ patients attending a memory clinic (Nuremberg, Germany) were diagnosed according to ICD-10 and tested with the SKT. The SKT consists of nine subtests, three for the assessment of memory and six for measuring attention in the sense of speed of information processing. The result of the SKT test procedure is a total score, which indicates the severity of overall cognitive impairment. Besides the summary score, two subscores for memory and attention can be interpreted. Using the level of depression as a covariate, statistical comparisons of SKT test profiles between the three patient groups revealed that depressed patients showed more pronounced deficits than MCI patients in all six attention subtests. On the other hand, MCI patients displayed significantly greater mnestic impairment than the depressed group, which was indicated by significant differences in the memory subscore. MCI and dementia patients showed similar deficit patterns dominated by impairment of memory (delayed recall) with MCI patients demonstrating less overall impairment. In sum, the SKT neuropsychological test profiles provided indicators for a differential diagnosis between MCI and beginning dementia vs. depression.

Keywords: differential diagnosis depression vs. MCI/dementia; mild cognitive impairment; dementia; depression in old age; SKT (Syndrom-Kurztest); cognitive assessment

1. Introduction

Dementia and depression are the most frequent psychiatric disorders of old age [1]. Both affect quality of life of patients in a more fundamental way and to a much greater extent than many somatic diseases [2]. Depression is also considered a serious risk factor for developing dementia [3,4]. In addition, dementia and depression share a diagnostic deficit. Dementia is often only diagnosed in more advanced stages showing higher degrees of functional impairment [5]. Worldwide, patients suffering from depression frequently are not correctly diagnosed; therefore, in many countries less than 10% of depressed subjects receive adequate treatment [6].

Due to an overlap in symptoms, a valid differential diagnosis between dementia and depression is sometimes difficult to establish: Depressive disorders in old age are associated with cognitive impairment in 40% to 60% of patients [7]. Conversely, about 40% of dementia patients develop depression symptoms [8,9]. Accordingly, among the differential diagnoses of dementia, in the first place the ICD-10 [10] lists depressive disorders, which can show characteristics of incipient dementia with memory impairment, slowed thinking and lack of spontaneity. In the same way, the DSM-5 [11] recommends inspecting the cognitive profiles of patients suggesting memory and executive impairment as typical for Alzheimer's disease, whereas nonspecific and more variable test performance could be expected in major depression. In accordance with this perspective, a number of reviews state a lack of clarity in the neuropsychological profiles of depressive disorders [12,13]. However, other authors consider impairment in speed of information processing, attention or executive functions as cognitive core features of depressed older patients [7,14–16].

Since the cognitive deficits associated with depression are less pronounced than those found in dementia [17–19], making a differential diagnosis much more difficult when it is not a full-blown dementia, but "mild cognitive impairment" (MCI), which has to be differentiated from depression. For almost 30 years, MCI has been conceptualized as a transitional phase between normal aging and dementia; it is discussed as a clinical condition with a high prognostic value for future dementia development, mostly towards Alzheimer's dementia [20–22]. The diagnostic differentiation of MCI and depression is further complicated by the existence of several MCI subtypes (amnestic vs. non-amnestic, single vs. multiple domains) causing a potential variety of neuropsychological performance patterns. Furthermore, nearly one third of MCI patients also will develop depression symptoms [23]. Overall, a wide range of disturbed cognitive functions may be expected in both MCI and depressed subjects. Consequently, attempts to differentiate between MCI and depression by means of psychometric tests often have failed [18,19,24].

Against this background, the present study compared the neuropsychological profiles of patients with MCI, mild dementia and depression tested with the SKT according to Erzigkeit [25]. The SKT (acronym for Syndrom-Kurztest; however, this German term is outdated and not used anymore) is a short cognitive performance test assessing memory and attention, the latter in the sense of speed of information processing. Thus, the SKT addresses exactly those two cognitive domains that are considered to be primarily impaired in patients with mild dementia and depressive disorders, respectively. Furthermore, given the fact that amnestic MCI is the most frequent MCI subtype [24,26], it was expected that patients with MCI or mild dementia would show greater deficits in the memory section of the SKT, while depressed patients would be more impaired in subtests measuring speed of information processing.

2. Methods

2.1. Samples

The present study included all patients referred between 2000 and 2005 to the Memory Clinic of Nuremberg General Hospital fulfilling the following criteria: (1) age 60 years or older, (2) diagnosis of mild cognitive impairment (MCI, in accordance with the consensus criteria according to Winblad et al. 2004 [20]), mild dementia (Alzheimer type, mixed type or vascular dementia; ICD-10 codes F00 or F01) or depressive disorder (ICD-10 codes F32 or F33) and (3) complete assessment with all SKT subtests. As an indicator of the clinical severity of MCI and mild dementia, assignment to stages 3 (MCI) or 4 (mild dementia) of the Global Deterioration Scale (GDS, [27]) was required. Exclusion criteria were (1) age below 60 years, (2) all other diagnoses than the ones required for inclusion, e.g., other forms of dementia (dementia in Parkinson disease and amnesic syndromes due to substance use), other forms of depression (e.g., adjustment disorders or post-traumatic stress disorders) and (3) not being able to complete all SKT subtests (e.g., due to reduced motor abilities, due to not being able to understand the test instructions or being unfamiliar with numbers).

2.2. Measures

The SKT is a cognitive test developed and published in Germany [28] assessing impairment of memory and attention, the latter in the sense of speed of information processing. The SKT comprises nine subtests, three of which refer to visual memory (immediate and delayed recall and recognition memory), the remaining six subtests measure processing speed. An overview of the subtests and the tasks to be completed is given in Table 1, the test materials are shown in Figure 1.

Table 1. Overview of the nine Syndrom-Kurztest (SKT) subtests.

Name of Subtest	Content of Subtest	Domain
I Naming Objects	twelve objects have to be named and memorized at the same time	attention/speed
II Immediate Recall	recall of objects shown in subtest I	memory
III Naming Numerals	two digit numbers written on magnetic blocks placed on a board have to be read out loud	attention/speed
IV Arranging Blocks	the magnetic blocks have to be arranged in ascending order of the numbers	attention/speed
V Replacing Blocks	the blocks have to be replaced in their original positions	attention/speed
VI Counting Symbols	symbols printed on a tableau have to be counted	attention/speed
VII Reversal Naming	two rows composed of two letters in random order are to be read by naming each letter with the name of the other	attention/speed
VIII Delayed Recall	recall of objects shown in subtest I	memory
IX Recognition Memory	identification of objects shown in subtest I from a table containing 48 objects	memory

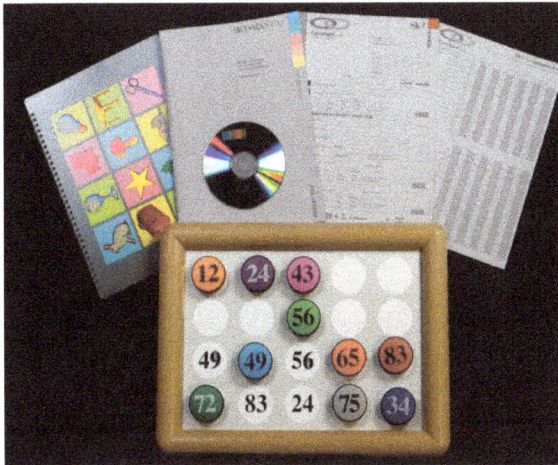

Figure 1. SKT test materials.

The maximum performance time for each subtest is limited to 60 s, so that the total administration time will be approximately 10 to 15 min. In the attention/speed subtests, the patient is instructed to work as fast and accurately as possible. In the memory subtests, all correct answers given within 60 s will be scored. The test was developed in five parallel forms (A to E) for repeated test administration even within short time intervals. In addition to a total summary score, the evaluation also provides subscores for separately interpreting memory and attention performance.

Since its publication in 1977, the SKT has been revised three times. The last revision carried out in 2015 was undertaken to establish new test norms for age groups 60 years and older to improve the sensitivity of the SKT for early cognitive decline due to Alzheimer's disease or other neurocognitive disorders [25]. In a first step, more than 1000 non-demented community dwelling subjects aged between 60 and 91 years were tested with the SKT. On the basis of this data set, conditional expected values were calculated for each of the nine SKT subtests using multiple regressions taking into account age, gender and level of intelligence. Based on the deviations from the predicted performance, in a second step, norm scores of 0, 1 or 2 were defined depending on the size of the deviation of the actual performance from the predicted performance (higher scores indicating greater cognitive impairment). The SKT total summary score ranging between 0 and 18 is obtained by adding the deviation scores (i.e., norm scores) of the nine subtests and is visualized in a traffic light system. Total scores between 0 and 4 indicate "age-appropriate cognitive performance" (green), scores between 5 and 10 points suggest "mild cognitive impairment" (MCI, yellow) and values between 11 and 18 substantiate a "suspicion of beginning dementia" (red). It must be noted that the SKT total summary score can be reliably interpreted in case of a homogeneous test profile, i.e., the memory and attention domain are affected to a similar extent. In case of profile heterogeneity, the summary scores should be interpreted with caution and the severity of impairment should also be assessed separately for the two domains.

Besides the SKT, the standard test battery of the Nuremberg Memory Clinic comprised the CERAD-NP [29] and two different depression scales [30,31]. Furthermore, relatives rated the patient using the Bayer-ADL scale to stage functional capacities [32] and the Neuropsychiatric Interview [33] to assess behavioral disturbances occurring in dementia. The diagnostic classification of a given patient was made taking into account information from different sources (anamnesis, medical examination, neuropsychology, everyday functioning, and neuroimaging or laboratory results).

2.3. Statistics

The raw scores of the nine SKT subtests were converted into norm scores using the EXCEL program "SKT-Analyser-v10.xlsm" [25]. From these, the subscores for memory and attention as well as the SKT total summary score were calculated by adding the corresponding subtest scores (SKT subscores and total summary score are also included in the program printout). Using one-way analyses of variance, differences in the nine subtests, the two subscores and the SKT total summary score were checked for statistical significance between the three study groups. Pairwise group comparisons were based on the Tukey test. A Bonferroni correction for multiple comparisons was not carried out, as the focus of the analyses presented here was on the comparative examination of test profiles and less on the detection of robust group differences. Comparisons of SKT profiles across the nine subtests and the memory and attention subscores were performed using multivariate analyses of variance for repeated measurements. To assess the effect of depression on SKT scores, Pearson correlation coefficients were computed between depression scores [30,31] and the SKT summary score, the SKT memory and attention subscores and the norm scores of the nine SKT subtests. Moreover, we repeated the analyses of variance controlling for depression to establish a "pure" metric of cognitive impairment unbiased by affective disturbances. While we used two different depression scores, we calculated the mean of the transformed z-scores [30,31]. Furthermore, a receiver operator characteristics (ROC) analysis was employed to compute areas under the curve (AUC) for each of the three diagnostic groups using the SKT norming sample comprising 1053 non-demented community dwelling subjects aged between 60 and 91 as a reference group. All analyses were carried out with the statistics program IBM SPSS Statistics (Version 20, Armonk, NY, United States) and were based on a completely anonymized data set. The study was registered in the study centre of the Nuremberg General Hospital as a quality assurance measure according to § 27/4 of the Bavarian Hospital Law.

3. Results

Of the 1362 patients assessed between 2000 and 2005 in the Nuremberg Memory Clinic, a total sample of $n = 549$ fulfilled the inclusion and exclusion criteria (see Section 2.1). The patients were distributed among the three diagnostic groups as follows: 172 patients were diagnosed with MCI, 166 patients were diagnosed with dementia (F00.0 or F00.1: 89 patients, F00.2: 39 patients and F01: 38 patients), 211 patients suffered from first manifested or recurrent depression (F32: 150 patients and F33:

61 patients). Diagnoses were based on ICD-10 [10]. Sociodemographic data and SKT results (subtests, subscores and SKT total score) of the three study groups were compiled together with the results of the group comparisons in Table 2. The SKT test profiles of the three study samples are depicted in Figure 2.

Table 2. Demographic data, Mini-Mental State Examination (MMSE) and depression scores, SKT norm scores for subtests I to IX, SKT subscores for memory and attention and SKT total score. Frequencies (sample size and gender) or mean values with standard deviations in brackets are given.

	MCI M (SD)	DEM M (SD)	DEP M (SD)	*p*	Group Comparisons
sample size	172	166	211		
age	73.9 (7.3)	76.6 (7.6)	72.5 (7.5)	0.000	DEP < MCI < DEM
gender (f/m)	90/82	102/64	134/77	0.045	
education *	12,0 (2,8)	11,3 (2,9)	11,4 (2,8)	*n.s.*	
MMSE **	26.5 (2.2)	22.6 (3.1)	26.2 (3.0)	0.000	DEM < MCI = DEP
depression (z-scores) ***	−0.42 (0.77)	−0.27 (0.81)	0.55 (1.04)	0.000	DEM = MCI, MCI < DEP, DEM < DEP
SKT I	0.70 (0.87)	1.17 (0.90)	0.91 (0.93)	0.000	MCI < (tend.) DEP < DEM
SKT II	0.92 (0.93)	1.64 (0,72)	0.78 (0.93)	0.000	MCI = DEP; DEP < DEM; MCI < DEM
SKT III	0.56 (0.83)	0.89 (0.95)	0.69 (0.90)	0.003	MCI = DEP; DEP = DEM; MCI < DEM
SKT IV	1.01 (0.96)	1.49 (0.84)	1.22 (0.94)	0.000	MCI < (tend.) DEP < DEM
SKT V	1.12 (0.95)	1.50 (0.81)	1.28 (0.91)	0.000	MCI = DEP; DEP < (tend.) DEM; MCI < DEM
SKT VI	0.67 (0.87)	0.99 (0.95)	0.91 (0.96)	0.009	MCI < DEP; DEP = DEM; MCI < DEM
SKT VII	1.06 (0.95)	1.39 (0.89)	1.25 (0.93)	0.005	MCI = DEP; DEP = DEM; MCI < DEM
SKT VIII	1.24 (0.92)	1.77 (0.60)	0.86 (0.94)	0.000	DEP < MCI < DEM
SKT IX	0.87 (0.99)	1.46 (0.89)	0.83 (0.99)	0.000	DEP = MCI; DEP < DEM; MCI < DEM
SKT memory	3.03 (1.85)	4.87 (1.44)	2.47 (2.06)	0.000	DEP < MCI < DEM
SKT attention	5.12 (3.58)	7.42 (3.37)	6.27 (3.95)	0.000	MCI < DEP < DEM
SKT sum score	8.15 (3.97)	12.28 (3.55)	8.74 (4.78)	0.000	MCI= DEP; DEP < DEM; MCI < DEM

Abbreviations: MCI: mild cognitive impairment, DEM: dementia, DEP depression; MMSE: Mini-Mental State Examination, f: female, m: male, tend.: statistical tendency (*p* < 0.10);. * 19 missing; ** 1 missing; *** 53 missing.

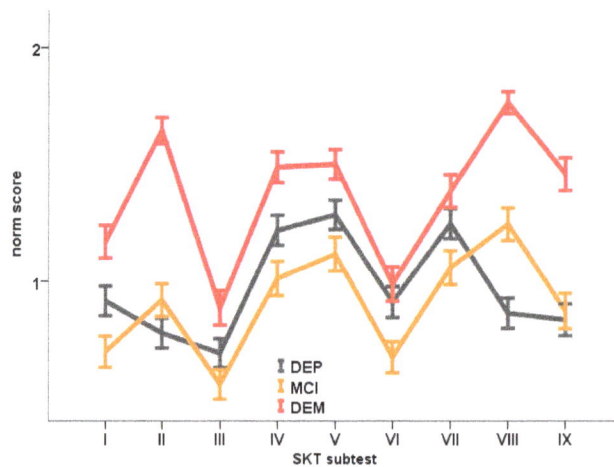

Figure 2. Norm scores (means) of the three study groups for the nine SKT subtests (I: naming objects, II: immediate recall, III: naming numerals, IV: arranging blocks, V: replacing blocks, VI: counting symbols, VII: reversal naming, VIII: delayed recall, IX: recognition memory).

As Figure 2 illustrates, the MCI and dementia group show peaks in their SKT profiles in subtest VIII, which examines the delayed recall of objects. In contrast, depressed patients reveal their most striking performance deficits in the speed subtests IV, V and VII. Furthermore, Figure 2 indicates less overall cognitive impairment in MCI and depressed subjects when compared to dementia patients. SKT total summary scores for the MCI and depressed groups displayed values between 8 and 9 points; they do not differ statistically between both groups (see Table 2). However, striking differences can be detected in their subtest profiles. While mean scores in memory subtests II, VIII and IX of MCI patients are consistently lower than those of subjects with dementia (level significance was reached for subtest VIII), depressed patients show more pronounced deficits than MCI patients in all six speed tests (with only the difference in subtest VI turned out to be significant, statistical tendencies ($p < 0.10$) were found for subtests I and IV). Subsequently, the memory subscore indicated significantly greater cognitive impairment in the MCI group and the attention subscore in the depression group ($p < 0.05$ each).

The comparison of the SKT profiles between the three diagnostic groups included in the study across all nine subtests revealed a highly significant interaction effect 'diagnosis × subtest' (Pillai's Trace = 0.121 with F (16, 1080) = 4.34, $p < 0.000$) in a multivariate analysis of variance with repeated measures (MANOVA), which indicates an overall difference of test profiles. Subsequent pairwise comparisons performed to identify the source of this interaction effect revealed a marginally non-significant interaction (Pillai's Trace = 0.045 with F (8, 329) = 1.59, p = 0.054) for the comparison MCI vs. dementia, indicating a relative similarity of the subtest profiles between these two groups. The two remaining contrasts, MCI vs. depression and dementia vs. depression, were again significant with respect to the interaction term 'diagnosis × subtest' (MCI vs. depression: Pillai's Trace = 0.066; F (8, 329) = 3.31, p < 0.001; depression vs. dementia: Pillai's Trace = 0.0148; F (8, 329) = 8.01, p < 0.000) pointing towards the depression group as the source of the overall difference between profiles.

More clearly than the profile comparisons across subtests, the comparison of the SKT memory and attention subscores revealed the different impairment patterns between diagnostic groups MCI/mild dementia vs. depression. When comparing the three subsamples, the interaction 'diagnosis × subscore' reached significance (Pillai's Trace = 0.034; F (2, 546) = 2.55, p < 0.000). However, when comparing only MCI vs. dementia, the level of significance was missed more clearly for the SKT subscore profile than for the subtest profile (Pillai's Trace = 0.004 with F (1, 336) = 1.18, p = 0.277). This result demonstrates the similarity of the SKT subscore profiles between MCI and mild dementia. The remaining comparisons

(MCI vs. depression and dementia vs. depression) again showed significant interaction effects, which can be interpreted in terms of different subtest compositions in MCI/mild dementia vs. depression (MCI vs. depression: Pillai's Trace = 0.042; F (1, 381) = 16.52, p < 0.000; dementia vs. depression: Pillai's Trace = 0.024; F (1, 375) = 9.18, p < 0.01).

Pearson correlation coefficients between SKT and depression scores ranged between r = −0.15–0.20 in the total sample and hardly exceeded r = 0.20 in the three subsamples (MCI: range *r* = 0.02–0.20; DEM: range *r* = −0.22–0.15; DEP: range *r* = −0.03–0.17). Accordingly, introducing depression as a covariate into the analyses of variance did not fundamentally change the outcome. Regarding significance, seven out of eight comparisons remained significant, even though less pronounced. Noteworthy, the differences in SKT subtest and subscore profiles between MCI vs. depression outlasted the correction for depression. When comparing these two groups, the interaction terms remained significant (diagnosis × subtest: Pillai's Trace = 0.046; F (8,351) = 2.130, p = 0.033; diagnosis × subscore: Pillai's Trace = 0.017; F (1,358) = 6.29, p = 0.013). Finally, Table 3 displays the results of the ROC analyses examining the ability of the SKT sum score and the subscores to correctly classify MCI, dementia and depression. All SKT scores were based on the SKT norming sample used for developing the regression based norms [25].

Table 3. Results of receiver operating curves (ROC): area under curve (AUC).

	MCI	DEM	DEP
SKT sum score	0.83	0.96	0.81
SKT memory subscore	0.77	0.93	0.68
SKT attention subscore	0.74	0.88	0.79

4. Discussion

In the present analyses, the newly-normed SKT, a short cognitive performance test for assessing deficits of memory and attention, revealed different neuropsychological profiles for patients belonging to the MCI/mild dementia spectrum on the one hand, and patients suffering from depressive disorders on the other. In the MCI and dementia conditions, the deficit patterns displayed their peaks for the delayed memory recall of objects. Since amnestic MCI (isolated or in combination with other cognitive domains) is considered to be the most frequent MCI subtype [24,26] and impaired episodic memory is a prerequisite for a dementia diagnosis according to the ICD-10 criteria, this result is not really surprising. However, it can be taken as an indication of the construct validity of the SKT as a tool to support diagnosis in organic mental disorders. It may be expected that the assessment of patients with other forms of dementia, e.g., Lewy-Body, Frontal Lobe or Parkinson's, might have resulted in different test profiles. In the same vein, an exploratory investigation comparing SKT subtest patterns of patients diagnosed with Alzheimer's and Parkinson's dementia using the old test norms [34] indicated greater impairment of Parkinson patients in subtests assessing speed of information processing with subtest V (replacing blocks) reaching the level of statistical significance. Moreover, the slowing of speed of information processing, especially in tasks with a strong executive component, which could be observed in the depressed sample of the study has been described as a characteristic neuropsychological feature of depression [7,14,15].

To address a common misunderstanding, it must be pointed out that the SKT is not a test exclusively for the area of dementia. Originally, it was developed for usage with patients older than 17 years of age suffering from acute or chronic mental disorders irrespective of their aetiology. Therefore, there is ample experience with the SKT in the cross-sectional and longitudinal assessment of cognitive impairment resulting, e.g., from brain injury, substance abuse or anesthesia [35]. The misclassification of the SKT as a dementia test was surely supported by the fact that the SKT has been used as an outcome measure in more than 50 studies investigating the efficacy of various nootropic compounds, cognition enhancers or antidementia drugs, in the past years with a clear focus on the efficacy of Ginkgo biloba [35].

In line with this shift of test usage towards dementing disorders starting in the 1980s, all three test revisions of the SKT focused on older patients suffering from cognitive impairment. The first modification in 1989 aimed at making test materials more appealing [36]. The second revision suggested a finer classification of age norms beyond the age of 65 and included an option for separate assessment of memory and speed functions allowing for differential diagnostic considerations [37]. Finally, the new norming of 2015 [25] served the purpose of improving the sensitivity of the test for early recognition of dementia in persons aged 60 years or older. First data show the high sensitivity and specificity of the SKT for dementia being 0.83 and 0.84, respectively [38,39]. The results of the ROC analyses reported in the present study support these findings.

Of special interest in the present investigation is the finding that the analysis of the SKT subscores for memory and attention revealed statistically significant differences between MCI and depressed patients. Other working groups, e.g., Barth et al. (2005) [18] using the CERAD-NP test battery did not find significant differences between MCI and depression in any of the CERAD tasks. In the same way, Zihl et al. (2010) [24] analyzing neuropsychological test data of MCI and cognitively impaired depressed patients also applying the CERAD-NP and an additional series of other psychometric instruments did not receive a single significant difference between both diagnostic groups. Nevertheless, they identified a significant reduction in speed of information processing for their depressed patients when comparing the results to cognitively normal older controls. This may be taken as a further indication that processing speed is a core domain affected by depression, which is in full accordance with the present results. Accordingly, our ROC analyses for depression vs. controls revealed a higher discriminative power of the SKT speed subscore in comparison to the memory subscore. Furthermore, the fact that the differences in SKT subscores for memory and speed performance outlasted a correction for (self-rated) depression may cautiously be considered as a hint of reduced speed of information processing as a trait marker for depression. This interpretation is supported by results that speed and executive test performance of depressed patients who were successfully treated was improved, but not normalized [15]. Finally, in a study by Dierckx et al. (2007) [19] a cued recall paradigm discriminated well between Alzheimer patients and depressed subjects, but considerably lost diagnostic accuracy for separating MCI from depression. The authors explain this finding by the heterogeneity among MCI patients and a diagnostic uncertainty induced by misdiagnosing MCI in the presence of affective symptoms as depression.

Differential diagnosis between MCI/dementia and depression is not only complicated by an overlap in cognitive and affective symptoms. Meanwhile, there is evidence that MCI/dementia and depression share common pathophysiological pathways (e.g., [40,41]). On the one hand, depression seems to play a role in the pathogenesis of Alzheimer's disease via stress and a glucocorticoid increase that may cause amyloid-beta production or hippocampal atrophy resulting in an elevated dementia risk in depressed subjects. On the other hand, neurodegenerative and cerebrovascular alterations in the brain are discussed as etiological factors of depression [42,43]. Thus, in the future it is desirable that the clinical and psychometric assessment of patients suffering from cognitive and/or affective symptoms should be supplemented by information available from biomarkers reflecting neuronal or vascular damage. This could allow for defining MCI [21] and depression subgroups bearing a higher risk for cognitive decline towards a dementia syndrome. The next step for our working group will be an analysis of SKT follow-up data that might be available for MCI and depressed patients participating in the present investigation to validate their diagnostic classifications.

A final remark refers to the international validity of the SKT, which up to about 1990 was mainly used in German-speaking countries. However, in the following years an increasing number of international studies were performed, e.g., in the United States, the UK, Greece, Russia, Chile, Mexico, Brazil or South Korea [44–50]. Some of these studies specifically aimed at validating the SKT for the respective target language or culture. To summarize a few findings, the transcultural transfer of the (mostly nonverbal) SKT test materials only required minor adjustments of some objects shown in subtest I (because they were less familiar in the target countries) or the adaptation of letters to be read in subtest VII (especially for countries using non-Latin letters). In many of these studies, the SKT kept the psychometric properties or factor structure comparable to the original German test version. However, the dependency of test results on education becomes critical especially with patients from developing countries with very few years of formal school education [47,49].

In 2019, the German standardization study of 2015, which established the new testing norms was replicated in three testing centers in the USA, Australia and Ireland with a somewhat smaller sample of altogether 285 cognitively unimpaired persons aged between 60 and 96 years [35,51]. As in the German study, the most important predictors of the SKT performance were age, age-squared, gender and intelligence. The explained variance was comparable to that found in the German standardization sample suggesting that the regression-based German SKT norms from 2015 are well matched by those found in 2019 for English speaking subjects. This equivalence may be taken as evidence for the cross-cultural stability of the SKT in German and English speaking countries of the Western world (see also [45]). It indicates that the SKT in its present form may be used without any further adaptations of the testing material in these regions. Taken together, the results of the present study confirm that the SKT can be considered as a neuropsychological test instrument validly assessing impairment in two cognitive domains, i.e., memory and attention (speed of information processing), which should always be addressed for a comprehensive diagnostic work-up within the spectrum of neurodevelopmental (ICD-11) or neurocognitive disorders (DSM-5).

Author Contributions: H.L. and M.S. wrote the manuscript; H.L. did all the statistical analyses.

Funding: This research received no external funding. The new standardization was supported by Willmar Schwabe Arzneimittel, Karlsruhe, Germany.

Acknowledgments: The article is dedicated to the memory of Hellmut Erzigkeit, who passed much too early in 2010. Hellmut Erzigkeit developed and published the SKT in the 1970s. For many years, he directed the Department of Clinical Psychology of the Psychiatric University Hospital Erlangen, Germany. Hartmut Lehfeld worked with him for many years. Hellmut Erzigkeit inspired many scientific projects, he was a visionary of psychometric assessment. We also deeply thank Robert Hoerr (Willmar Schwabe Arzneimittel, Karlsruhe, Germany) for his valuable comments and for proof reading the manuscript and Sophia Schneider (University of Erlangen-Nuremberg, Germany) for completing and correcting the reference list.

Conflicts of Interest: Mark Stemmler and Hartmut Lehfeld worked together in planning, running and evaluating the new standardization of the SKT and contributed significantly to the revised test manuals available in German and English. Hartmut Lehfeld receives royalty fees from the holder of the test's copyrights (Geromed GmbH, Spardorf). Mark Stemmler received fees from Geromed GmbH for scientific advice.

References

1. Wernicke, T.F.; Linden, M.; Gilberg, R.; Helmchen, H. Ranges of psychiatric morbidity in the old and the very old–results from the Berlin Aging Study (BASE). *Eur. Arch. Psychiatry Clin. Neurosci.* **2000**, *250*, 111–119. [CrossRef] [PubMed]

2. Murray, C.J.L.; Vos, T.; Lozano, R.; Mohsen, N.; Flaxman, A.D.; Michaud, C.; Ezzati, M.; Shibuya, K.; Salomon, J.A.; Abdalla, S.; et al. Disability-adjusted life years (DALYs) for 291 diseases and injuries in 21 regions, 1990–2010: A systematic analysis for the global burden of disease study 2010. *Lancet* **2012**, *380*, 2197–2223. [CrossRef]

3. Barnes, D.; Yaffe, K.; Byers, A.L.; McCormick, M.; Schaefer, C.; Whitmer, R. Midlife vs Late-Life Depressive Symptoms and Risk of Dementia Differential Effects for Alzheimer Disease and Vascular Dementia. *Arch. Gen. Psychiatry* **2012**, *69*, 493–498. [PubMed]

4. Singh-Manoux, A.; Dugravot, A.; Fournier, A.; Abell, J.; Ebmeier, K.; Kivimäki, M.; Sabia, S. Trajectories of Depressive Symptoms Before Diagnosis of Dementia: A 28-Year Follow-up Study. *JAMA Psychiatry* **2017**. [CrossRef] [PubMed]

5. Amjad, H.; Roth, D.L.; Sheehan, O.C.; Lyketsos, C.G.; Wolff, J.L.; Samus, Q.M. Underdiagnosis of Dementia: An Observational Study of Patterns in Diagnosis and Awareness in US Older Adults. *J. Gen. Intern. Med.* **2018**, *33*, 1131–1138. [CrossRef]

6. Depression: Fact sheet. Available online: https://www.who.int/news-room/fact-sheets/detail/depression (accessed on 7 July 2019).

7. Dybedal, G.S.; Tanum, L.; Sundet, K.; Gaarden, T.L.; Bjølseth, T.M. Neuropsychological functioning in late-life depression. *Front. Psychol.* **2013**, *4*, 381. [CrossRef]

8. Mega, M.S.; Cummings, J.L.; Fiorello, T.; Gornbein, J. The spectrum of behavioral changes in Alzheimer's disease. *Neurology* **1996**, *46*, 130–135. [CrossRef]

9. Zhao, Q.-F.; Tan, L.; Wang, H.-F.; Jiang, T.; Tan, M.-S.; Tan, L.; Xu, W.; Li, J.Q.; Wang, J.; Lai, T.J.; et al. The prevalence of neuropsychiatric symptoms in Alzheimer's disease: Systematic review and meta-analysis. *J. Affect. Disord.* **2016**, *190*, 264–271. [CrossRef]

10. Dilling, H.; Mombour, W.; Schmidt, M.H.; Schulte-Markwort, M. *Weltgesundheitsorganisation: Internationale Klassifikation psychischer Störungen: ICD-10 Kapitel V (F). Diagnostische Kriterien für Forschung und Praxis*, 3rd ed.; Verlag Hans Huber: Toronto, ON, Canada, 1999; pp. 181–183.

11. APA American Psychiatric Association. *Diagnostic and Statistical Manual of Mental Disorders (DSM-5®)*; American Psychiatric Pub: Washington, DC, USA, 2013.

12. Lee, R.S.; Hermens, D.F.; Porter, M.A.; Redoblado-Hodge, M.A. A meta-analysis of cognitive deficits in first-episode major depressive disorder. *J. Affect. Disord.* **2012**, *140*, 113–124. [CrossRef]

13. Beblo, T.; Sinnamon, G.; Baune, B.T. Specifying the neuropsychology of affective disorders: Clinical, demographic and neurobiological factors. *Neuropsychol. Rev.* **2011**, *21*, 337–359. [CrossRef]

14. Butters, M.A.; Whyte, E.M.; Nebes, R.D.; Begley, A.E.; Dew, M.A.; Mulsant, B.H.; Zmuda, M.D.; Bhalla, R.; Meltzer, C.C.; Pollock, B.G.; et al. The nature and determinants of neuropsychological functioning in late-life depression. *Arch. Gen. Psychiatry.* **2004**, *61*, 587–595. [CrossRef] [PubMed]

15. Gualtieri, C.T.; Johnson, L.G.; Benedict, K.B. Neurocognition in depression: Patients on and off medication versus healthy comparison subjects. *J. Neuropsychiatry Clin. Neurosci.* **2016**, *18*, 217–225. [CrossRef] [PubMed]

16. Rock, P.L.; Roiser, J.P.; Riedel, W.J.; Blackwell, A.D. Cognitive impairment in depression: A systematic review and meta-analysis. *Psychol. Med.* **2014**, *44*, 2029–2040. [CrossRef] [PubMed]

17. Künig, G.; Jäger, M.; Stief, V.; Kaldune, A.; Urbaniok, F.; Endrass, J. The impact of the CERAD-NP on diagnosis of cognitive deficiencies in late onset depression and Alzheimer's disease. *Int. J. Geriatr. Psychiatry.* **2006**, *21*, 911–916. [CrossRef]

18. Barth, S.; Schönknecht, P.; Pantel, J.; Schröder, J. Neuropsychologische Profile in der Demenzdiagnostik: Eine Untersuchung mit der CERAD-NP-Testbatterie. [Mild Cognitive Impairment and Alzheimer's Disease: An Investigation of the CERAD–NP Test Battery. *Fortschr. Der. Neurol. Und. Der. Psychiatr* **2005**, *73*, 568–576. [CrossRef]

19. Dierckx, E.; Engelborghs, S.; Raedt, R.D.; Deyn, P.P.D.; Ponjaert-Kristoffersen, I. Differentiation between mild cognitive impairment, Alzheimer's disease and depression by means of cued recall. *Psychol. Med.* **2007**, *37*, 747–755. [CrossRef]

20. Winblad, B.; Palmer, K.; Kivipelto, M.; Jelic, V.; Fratiglioni, L.; Wahlund, L.O.; Nordberg, A.; Bäckman, L.; Albert, M.; Almkvist, O.; et al. Mild cognitive impairment–beyond controversies, towards a consensus: Report of the International Working Group on Mild Cognitive Impairment. *J. Intern. Med.* **2004**, *256*, 240–246. [CrossRef]

21. Albert, M.S.; DeKosky, S.T.; Dickson, D.; Dubois, B.; Feldman, H.H.; Fox, N.C.; Gamst, A.; Holtzman, D.M.; Jagust, W.J.; Petersen, R.C.; et al. The diagnosis of mild cognitive impairment due to Alzheimer's disease: Recommendations from the National Institute on Aging-Alzheimer's Association workgroups on diagnostic guidelines for Alzheimer's disease. *Alzheimer's. Dis. Dement.* **2011**, *7*, 270–279. [CrossRef]

22. Petersen, R.C.; Caracciolo, B.; Brayne, C.; Gauthier, S.; Jelic, V.; Fratiglioni, L. Mild cognitive impairment: A concept in evolution. *J. Intern. Med.* **2014**, *275*, 214–228. [CrossRef]

23. Ismail, Z.; Elbayoumi, H.; Fischer, C.E.; Hogan, D.B.; Millikin, C.P.; Schweizer, T.; Mortby, M.E.; Smith, E.E.; Patten, S.B.; Fiest, K.M. Prevalence of depression in patients with mild cognitive impairment: A systematic review and meta-analysis. *JAMA Psychiatry* **2017**, *74*, 58–67. [CrossRef]

24. Zihl, J.; Reppermund, S.; Thum, S.; Unger, K. Neuropsychological profiles in MCI and in depression: Differential cognitive dysfunction patterns or similar final common pathway disorder? *J. Psychiatr. Res.* **2010**, *44*, 647–654. [CrossRef] [PubMed]

25. Stemmler, M.; Lehfeld, H.; Horn, R. *SKT Manual Edition 2015*; Geromed GmbH: Spardorf, Bavaria, Germany, 2015.

26. Roberts, R.O.; Geda, Y.E.; Knopman, D.S.; Cha, R.H.; Pankratz, V.S.; Boeve, B.F.; Tangalos, E.G.; Ivnik, R.J.; Rocca, W.A.; Petersen, R.C. The incidence of MCI differs by subtype and is higher in men: The Mayo Clinic Study of Aging. *Neurology* **2012**, *78*, 342–351. [CrossRef] [PubMed]

27. Reisberg, B.; Ferris, S.H.; de Leon, M.J.; Crook, T. The Global Deterioration Scale for assessment of primary degenerative dementia. *Am. J. Psychiatry* **1982**, *139*, 1136–1139. [PubMed]

28. Erzigkeit, H. *Manual for the Syndrom-Kurztest*; Geromed GmbH: Spardorf, Germany, 1997.

29. Monsch, A. *CERAD—Neuropsychological Test Battery*; Memory Clinic: Basel, Switzerland, 1997.

30. Hautzinger, M.; Bailer, M. *ADS, General Depression Scale*; Hogrefe Publishing GmbH: Göttingen, Germany, 1993.

31. Collegium Internationale Psychiatriae Scalarum (Hrsg.). *International Scales for Psychiatry*, 5th ed; Hogrefe Publishing GmbH: Göttingen, Germany, 2005.

32. Hindmarch, I.; Lehfeld, H.; de Jongh, P.; Erzigkeit, H. The Bayer Activities of Daily Living Scale (B-ADL Scale). *Dement. Geriatr. Cogn. Disord.* **1998**, *9*, 20–26. [CrossRef] [PubMed]

33. Cummings, J.L.; Mega, M.; Gray, K.; Rosenberg-Thompson, S.; Carusi, D.A.; Gornbein, J. The Neuropsychiatric Inventory: Comprehensive assessment of psychopathology in dementia. *Neurology* **1994**, *44*, 2308–2314. [CrossRef] [PubMed]

34. Stroessenreuther, N.; Lehfeld, H.; Niklewski, N. PANDA—A screening tool Parkinson neuropsychometric dementia assessment. In Proceedings of the DGPPN Congress, Berlin, Germany, 24–27 November 2010.

35. Stemmler, M.; Lehfeld, H.; Erzigkeit, A. The English Validation of the SKT according to Erzigkeit. In *SKT Manual Edition 2019*; Geromed GmbH: Spardorf, Bavaria, Germany, 2019.

36. Erzigkeit, H. *Manual for the SKT forms A-E*, 4th ed.; Beltz: Weinheim, Germany, 1989.

37. Lehfeld, H.; Erzigkeit, H. The SKT—A short cognitive performance test for assessing deficits of memory and attention. *Int. Psychogeriatr.* **1997**, *9*, 115–121. [CrossRef]

38. Hessler, J.B.; Stemmler, M.; Bickel, H. Cross-Validation of the newly-normed SKT for the detection of MCI and dementia. *GeroPsych.* **2017**, *30*, 19–25. [CrossRef]

39. Stemmler, M.; Hessler, J.B.; Bickel, H. Predicting cognitive decline and dementia with the newly-normed SKT Short Cognitive Performance Test. *Dement. Geriatr. Cogn. Disord. Extra* **2019**, *9*, 184–193. [CrossRef]

40. Butters, M.A.; Young, J.B.; Lopez, O.; Aizenstein, H.J.; Mulsant, B.H.; Reynolds III, C.F.; DeKosky, S.T.; Becker, J.T. Pathways linking late-life depression to persistent cognitive impairment and dementia. *Dialogues Clin. Neurosci.* **2008**, *10*, 345–357.

41. Wang, L.; Potter, G.G.; Krishnan, R.K.; Dolcos, F.; Smith, G.S.; Steffens, D.C. Neural correlates associated with cognitive decline in late-life depression. *Am. J. Geriatr Psychiatry* **2012**, *20*, 653–663. [CrossRef]

42. Aizenstein, H.J.; Baskys, A.; Boldrini, M.; Butters, M.A.; Diniz, B.S.; Jaiswal, M.K.; Jellinger, K.A.; Kruglov, L.S.; Meshandin, I.A.; Mijajlovic, M.D.; et al. Vascular depression consensus report—A critical update. *Bmc Med.* **2016**, *14*, 161. [CrossRef] [PubMed]

43. Yatawara, C.; Lee, D.; Ng, K.P.; Chander, R.; Ng, D.; Ji, F.; Shim, H.Y.; Hilal, S.; Venketasubramanian, N.; Chen, C.; et al. Mechanisms Linking White Matter Lesions, Tract Integrity and Depression in Alzheimer's Disease. *Am. J. Geriatr. Psychiatry* **2019**. [CrossRef] [PubMed]

44. Kim, Y.S.; Nibbelink, D.W.; Overall, J.E. Factor structure and scoring of the SKT test battery. *J. Clin. Psychol.* **1993**, *49*, 61–71. [CrossRef]

45. Lehfeld, H.; Rudinger, G.; Rietz, C.; Heinrich, C.; Wied, V.; Fornazzari, L.; Pittas, J.; Hindmarch, I.; Erzigkeit, H. Evidence of the cross-cultural stability of the factor structure of the SKT short test for assessing deficits of memory and attention. *Int. Psychogeriatr.* **1997**, *9*, 139–153. [CrossRef] [PubMed]

46. Tsolakis, M.; Pittas, J. The use of SKT for the assessment of dementia in Greece. *Encephalos* **1995**, *32*, 336–345.

47. Flaks, M.K.; Forlenza, O.V.; Pereira, F.S.; Viola, L.F.; Yassuda, M.S. Short cognitive performance test: Diagnostic accuracy and education bias in older Brazilian adults. *Arch. Clin. Neuropsychol.* **2009**, *24*, 301–306. [CrossRef] [PubMed]

48. Fornazzari, L.; Cumsille, F.; Quevedo, F.; Quiroga, P.; Rioseco, P.; Klaasen, G.; Martinez, C.G.; Rhode, G.; Sacks, C.; Rivera, E.; et al. Spanish validation of the Syndrom Kurztest (SKT). *Alzheimer Dis. Assoc. Disord.* **2001**, *15*, 211–215. [CrossRef]

49. Ostrosky-Solís, F.; Davila, G.; Ortiz, X.; Vega, F.; Garcia Ramos, G.; de Celis, M.; Dávila, L.; Gómez, C.; Jiménez, S.; Juárez, S.; et al. Determination of normative criteria and validation of the SKT for use in Spanish-speaking populations. *Int. Psychogeriatr.* **1999**, *11*, 171–180. [CrossRef]

50. Choi, S.H.; Lee, B.H.; Hahm, D.S.; Jeong, J.H.; Ha, C.K.; Han, S.H.; Erzigkeit, H.; Na, D.L. Validation of the Korean version of the Syndrom Kurztest (SKT): A short test for the assessment of memory and attention. *Hum. Psychopharmacol.* **2004**, *19*, 495–501. [CrossRef]

51. Stemmler, M.; Lehfeld, H. Validation of the SKT short cognitive performance test for the detection of early cognitive decline in English-speaking countries. In Proceedings of the CTAD Conference, San Diego CA, USA, 4–7 December 2019.

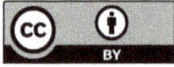

diagnostics

MDPI

Article

Who Is Classified as Untestable on Brief Cognitive Screens in an Acute Stroke Setting?

Emma Elliott *, Bogna A. Drozdowska, Martin Taylor-Rowan, Robert C. Shaw, Gillian Cuthbertson and Terence J. Quinn

Institute of Cardiovascular and Medical Sciences, University of Glasgow, New Lister Building, Glasgow Royal Infirmary, Glasgow G31 2ER, UK
* Correspondence: e.elliott.2@research.gla.ac.uk

Received: 30 June 2019; Accepted: 12 August 2019; Published: 14 August 2019

Abstract: Full completion of cognitive screening tests can be problematic in the context of a stroke. Our aim was to examine the completion of various brief cognitive screens and explore reasons for untestability. Data were collected from consecutive stroke admissions (May 2016–August 2018). The cognitive assessment was attempted during the first week of admission. Patients were classified as partially untestable ($\geq$1 test item was incomplete) and fully untestable (where assessment was not attempted, and/or no questions answered). We assessed univariate and multivariate associations of test completion with: age (years), sex, stroke severity (National Institutes of Health Stroke Scale (NIHSS)), stroke classification, pre-morbid disability (modified Rankin Scale (mRS)), previous stroke and previous dementia diagnosis. Of 703 patients admitted (mean age: 69.4), 119 (17%) were classified as fully untestable and 58 (8%) were partially untestable. The 4A-test had 100% completion and the clock-draw task had the lowest completion (533/703, 76%). Independent associations with fully untestable status had a higher NIHSS score (odds ratio (OR): 1.18, 95% CI: 1.11–1.26), higher pre-morbid mRS (OR: 1.28, 95% CI: 1.02–1.60) and pre-stroke dementia (OR: 3.35, 95% CI: 1.53–7.32). Overall, a quarter of patients were classified as untestable on the cognitive assessment, with test incompletion related to stroke and non-stroke factors. Clinicians and researchers would benefit from guidance on how to make the best use of incomplete test data.

Keywords: feasibility; cognitive screening instruments; cognition; stroke

1. Introduction

Cognitive screening following a stroke is recommended in international clinical guidelines [1,2] and routinely performed in acute stroke settings in many countries. However, completion of a cognitive test battery in a medically unwell person with recent neurological insult is challenging. Previous research has demonstrated that around 20% of stroke patients cannot fully complete many of the cognitive screening tests commonly used in stroke practice, for example the Montreal Cognitive Assessment (MoCA) [3] and the Mini-Mental State Examination (MMSE) [4]. Test non-completion is reported in both acute stroke [5] and rehabilitation settings [6] (Table 1). However, published data appear conflicting and other centres have reported that a lengthy neuropsychological battery can be performed in the acute setting [7].

Table 1. Previous studies addressing feasibility of cognitive assessments post-stroke.

Study	Test	Number of Patients	Inclusion Criteria Relevant to Feasibility	Time Point	Completion Rate
Setting: Acute					
Alderman et al. [8] (CA)	Battery of 8 tests	27	Mild strokes and TIAs	≤24 h	96%
Collas 2016 [9] (CA)	OCS	155	No relevant exclusions	5 days (mean)	89%
Horstmann et al. [10]	MoCA	842	IS and ICH. No relevant exclusions	2 days (median)	81%
Pasi et al. [5]	MoCA	137	IS and ICH. No relevant exclusions	5–9 days	83%
Pendlebury et al. [11]	AMT MMSE	1097	No relevant exclusions	4 days (median)	76% partially testable 69% fully testable
Van Zandvoort et al. [7]	1.5-h NPB	57	IS only, no previous stroke, maximum age 80, mRS 2–4, no psychiatric history or comorbidity that could influence cognitive functioning	4–22 days	75%
Setting: Sub-Acute/Rehabilitation					
Barnay et al. [12]	CASP MMSE MoCA	44	All aphasic patients	42 ± 22 days	CASP 82% MMSE 64% MoCA 70%
Benaim et al. [6]	CASP MMSE MoCA	50	Non-aphasic patients only	40 ± 17 days	CASP 100% MMSE 100% MoCA 94%
Cumming et al. [13]	MoCA	220	IS and ICH. No relevant exclusions	3 months	Mild stroke 87% Moderate stroke 79% Severe stroke 67%
Kwa et al. [14]	CAMCOG	129	IS only	≥3 months	88%
Mancuso et al. [15]	OCS MMSE	325	No previous stroke, able to consent themselves, no previous psychiatric/neurological disease	33.9 ± 41.8 days	Fully untestable: MMSE 2%, OCS 1% Highest incompletion for individual OCS tasks: trails 28/325 (9%)
Lees et al. [16]	ACE-III MMSE MoCA	51	No relevant exclusions	36 days (median)	ACE-III 27% MMSE 43% MoCA 39%

Abbreviations: Abbreviated Mental Test (AMT); Addenbrooke's Cognitive Examination III (ACE-III); Cambridge Cognition Examination (CAMCOG); Cognitive assessment scale for stroke patients (CASP); conference abstract (CA); ischaemic stroke (IS); intracerebral haemorrhage (ICH); Mini-Mental State Examination (MMSE); Montreal Cognitive Assessment (MoCA); neuropsychological battery (NPB); Oxford Cognitive Screen (OCS); transient ischaemic attack (TIA); modified Rankin Scale (mRS).

Feasibility of completing a cognitive assessment is multifactorial; some aspects may relate to the stroke (extent of damage, presence of aphasia, limb weakness) and others may relate to the nature of the testing (timing and length of assessment, complexity). Looking at the patient characteristics and approaches to assessment can explain the apparently contradictory findings in the literature. Patients included in studies of cognitive tests are often not representative of a typical stroke unit. For example, studies may favour the inclusion of those with minor strokes, no (or little) pre-stroke disability and those who are able to provide informed consent, whilst patients with severe aphasia or an existing diagnosis of dementia are often excluded [17]. This selection bias will underestimate the true incidence of untestable patients.

An incomplete cognitive test has clinical implications. Inexperienced assessors may erroneously ascribe an incomplete test to cognitive impairment, when in the context of stroke, non-completion may relate to physical impairments. Ultimately, test non-completion could risk false positive and false negative diagnosis of cognitive problems with attendant harm. An understanding of the extent of test non-completion and knowledge of factors relating to untestability could potentially avoid this. The issue of test incompletion also complicates stroke research and audit. Often patients with incomplete assessments are excluded from analyses (since a total score cannot be calculated). This practice biases results, underestimates levels of cognitive impairment and could also lead to erroneous results [11]. Various approaches to incorporate incomplete tests have been proposed but there is no consensus on the best method [16].

There are different ways to address these feasibility issues, but the approach taken will depend on the aspect of feasibility of greatest relevance. For example, one may decide to choose a test specifically designed for a stroke (e.g., Oxford Cognitive Screen (OCS) [18]). This approach recognises that many traditional cognitive tests were designed for memory clinic populations and are not suited to the specific challenges encountered in acute stroke settings. Stroke specific, multi-domain tests are described and may be less biased by physical, communication and visuospatial impairments. Another approach may be to choose a shorter cognitive screen. This approach may be particularly suited to the acute medical setting where clinicians have limited time and other investigations may be prioritised in the first few days. Shorter tests may also be attractive to patients as there will be a reduced test burden. Short cognitive screens have been largely ignored in research conducted in the stroke setting. Stroke care is continuously evolving and differs internationally, but there is currently a paucity of feasibility research on cognitive tests in an acute, National Health Service (NHS) context. Our research aimed to meet these two gaps.

Our primary aim was to describe the test completion (feasibility) of some of the shortest cognitive screens (deliverable in under five min) in an unselected group admitted to our hyper-acute stroke unit. Our secondary aims were to explore reasons for assessors giving a patient a label of being untestable and to describe factors associated with being untestable.

2. Methods

We conducted an observational, cross-sectional study, using routinely collected data from an urban UK, teaching hospital. This was approved by the West of Scotland Research Ethics Committee (ws/16/0001) on 4 February 2016. We followed Standards of Reporting of Neurological Disorders (STROND) guidance [19] for the design, conduct and reporting of the study.

2.1. Setting and Population

We collected anonymised, routine, clinical data from consecutive admissions to our hyper-acute stroke unit (HASU). The unit admits all suspected stroke and transient ischaemic attack (TIA) patients with no exclusions in relation to age, disability or comorbidity. The unit offers level two (high dependency) clinical care and only patients requiring multi-organ support would be admitted to a higher-level care facility. Recruitment occurred during four timepoints: May 2016–February 2017; April–June 2017; October–December 2017; and July–August 2018. For the purposes of this study, we made no exclusions around stroke severity or stroke-related impairments. Written informed consent was not required for assessment.

2.2. Clinical and Demographic Assessment

Clinical and demographic data were collected for each patient by five trained researchers (four postgraduate students in psychology/neuroscience and one undergraduate medical student). Data collected were a mix of prospective assessment and retrospective derivation from medical case notes. Stroke severity was determined by the National Institutes of Health Stroke Scale (NIHSS) [20] on admission. Medical history, including any pre-stroke diagnosis of dementia, was recorded using medical notes and primary care summary data. Pre-stroke functioning was established using the modified Rankin Scale (mRS) [21–23]. Bamford stroke classification was completed for both ischaemic and haemorrhagic patients.

2.3. Cognitive Assessment

The cognitive assessment consisted of 13 questions, covering 8 different cognitive screening tests: the 10-point Abbreviated mental test score (AMTS) [24] and its shorter version AMT-4 [25], General Practitioner Assessment of Cognition (GPCOG) (patient section) [26], Mini-Cog [27], six item cognitive impairment test (6-CIT) [28], National Institute Neurological Disorders S-Canadian Stroke Network (NINDS-CSN) 5-min MoCA [29], abbreviated MoCA [30], and the 4 'A's Test (4AT) (Available online: www.the4AT.com) (Table 2). Each of these individual tests can be administered in under 5 min (and so suitable for use in acute clinical practice). They cover a variety of cognitive domains and have some supporting validation work in primary and geriatric care [31].

Table 2. Short cognitive tests ordered by number of items.

Test Name	Number of Items		Questions	Maximum Score	% of Assessments We Could Score in Full
Mini-Cog [27]	2	1	3-word delayed recall	5	75%
		2	Clock draw (numbers, hands)		
Abbreviated MoCA [30]	2	1	5-word delayed recall	8	75%
		2	Clock draw (face, numbers, hands)		
4-AMT [25]	4	1	Age	4	81%
		2	Year		
		3	Place		
		4	Date of birth		
4AT (Available online: www.the4AT.com)	5	1	Alertness	12	100%
		2	Age		
		3	Current year		
		4	Place		
		5	Date of birth		
		6	Months backwards		
6-CIT [28]	6	1	Time	28	78%
		2	Month		
		3	Yearl		
		4	Count backwards from 20		
		5	5-part delayed recall		
		6	Months backwards		
GPCOG [26]	7	1	Date	9	75%
		2	Month		
		3	Year		
		4	Date of birth		
		5	5-part delayed recall		
		6	Clock draw (numbers, hands)		
		7	News item		
NINDS-CSN 5 min MoCA [29]	7	1	Date	12	79%
		2	Month		
		3	Year		
		4	Day		
		5	Place		
		6	City		
		7	5-word delayed recall		
		8	Fluency (letter F)		
10-AMT [24]	10	1	Age	10	79%
		2	Time		
		3	Year		
		4	Place		
		5	Two-person recognition		
		6	Date of birth		
		7	Year of WW1		
		8	Current prime minister		
		9	Count backwards from 20		
		10	3-part delayed recall		

Abbreviations: Abbreviated mental test (AMT); General Practitioner Assessment of Cognition (GPCOG); Montreal Cognitive Assessment (MoCA); National Institute of Neurological disorders and stroke and the Canadian stroke network (NINDS-CSN); Six item cognitive impairment test (6-CIT).

Assessment was attempted during the first week of admission. Patients were only approached once for assessment, unless the patient requested for the assessment to be done at a later time-point, the assessment was interrupted by another clinical investigation (e.g., scan) or if the patient requested the assessment to be done over two sessions. Patients were not approached at all (and categorised fully untestable) if the parent clinical team reported that the patient was too unwell to undergo assessment or if the assessor felt that any form of direct testing would not be possible. In these patients, who could not be directly assessed, we checked if a cognitive assessment was documented by the parent clinical team since admission.

2.4. Defining the Test Completion Outcomes

Patients were classified as fully untestable when no part of the assessment was attempted (decision made by researcher in consultation with parent clinical team) and/or when no questions were answered when testing was attempted. Partially untestable was defined when at least one item in a test could not be completed or was not attempted (decided by either the patient, parent clinical team or researcher). A list of potential categories was created by the authors based on clinical experience, previous literature and initial scoping of free text responses. The free text reasons documented for each patient classified as untestable by the individual assessor were later collated into categories (e.g., aphasia and dysarthria both captured under speech problems) by the lead author (E.Elliott) with discussion with the stroke consultant (T.Quinn). Where more than one reason was listed, we chose the primary factor deemed to have the greatest impact on assessment (e.g., a patient documented as both acutely confused and dysarthric was categorised under confusion). Cases where a test item was attempted but poorly completed, for example, a patient with limb weakness who attempted the clock-draw with their weak or non-dominant hand, were classed as testable.

2.5. Statistical Analysis

We described patients as fully or partially untestable using the definitions above. We looked at the completion rate of each question in our assessment and then calculated completion rates for the different tests. Patients who ended up with a non-stroke diagnosis were kept in the analyses as we were interested in the feasibility of tests within all patients admitted with a suspected stroke and we retained admission NIHSS for these patients where it was completed.

We assessed univariable and multivariable associations with outcomes of interest using logistic regression. Variables were chosen based on previous literature [10,11] and plausible associations with feasibility. The following 12 covariates were used in both univariate and multivariate analyses: age (years), sex, NIHSS, Bamford stroke classification (TIA, partial anterior circulation stroke—PACS, total anterior circulation stroke—TACS, posterior circulation stroke—POCS, lacunar stroke—LACS, non-stroke (used as reference group)), pre-morbid mRS, presence of intracerebral haemorrhage (ICH), previous diagnosis of dementia and previous TIA/stroke. We did not include delirium in the model since our only measure was the 4AT scale and all untestable patients would have ended up with a label of delirium. Associations were described as odds ratios (OR) with corresponding 95% confidence intervals. We used the rule of 10 outcome events per predictor variable to determine the number of covariates we could include in the model and so required 120 "cases" for the model.

Analyses were run twice to account for how partially untestable patients are treated differently in the literature; in the first analysis they were treated as testable and in the second treated as untestable (grouped with the fully untestable patients). All data analyses were performed using the statistical software package SPSS (version 25 IBM, Armonk, NY, USA).

3. Results

The full sample included 703 patients (mean age 69.4 ± 13.7, 382 (54%) males, median NIHSS 2 (interquartile range, IQR 1–5)) (Table 3 for full patient characteristics). Of these, 119 (17%) were classified as fully untestable on all tests. Reasons for fully untestable fell under eight categories but for more than half of the group this was due to neurological deterioration (e.g., patients who were unresponsive, very unwell, palliative) (62/119, 54%). A further 58 (8%) patients in the full sample were separately classified as partially untestable (did not attempt ≥1 question); reasons fell under nine categories, with limb weakness 15 (26%) and speech problems 13 (22%) being most prevalent (full breakdown of reasons detailed in Figure 1). A large proportion of patients in the fully untestable group (*n* = 50, 42%) had a TACS, compared to only 3 (5%) in the partially untestable group.

Table 3. Characteristics of the sample.

Characteristics	Full Sample (*n* = 703)	Partially Untestable (*n* = 58)	Fully Untestable (*n* = 119)
Sex (male)	382 (54%)	27 (47%)	59 (50%)
Age mean (SD)	69.4 (13.7) Missing data (*n* = 2)	76.6 (9.7)	76.8 (12.5) Missing data (*n* = 2)
IS ICH TIA Non-stroke	429 IS 22 ICH 137 TIA 109 N/S Missing data (*n* = 6)	42 IS 4 ICH 5 TIA 7 N/S	85 IS 8 ICH 11 TIA 13 N/S Missing data (*n* = 2)
Bamford classification (IS and ICH)	66 TACS 174 PACS 100 POCS 111 LACS Missing data (*n* = 6)	3 TACS 25 PACS 12 POCS 6 LACS	50 TACS 31 PACS 8 POCS 4 LACS Missing data (*n* = 2)
NIHSS median (IQR)	2 (1–5) Missing data (*n* = 15)	4 (3–7) Missing data (*n* = 1)	8 (4–16) Missing data (*n* = 2)
Pre-morbid mRS median (IQR)	1 (0–3) Missing data (*n* = 5)	2 (0–3)	3 (0–3) Missing data (*n* = 1)
Previous stroke (IS/ICH) or TIA (yes)	218 (31%)	20 (34%)	36 (30%)
Previous diagnosis of dementia (yes)	61 (9%)	8 (14%)	30 (25%)

Abbreviations: ischaemic stroke (IS); interquartile range (IQR); intracerebral haemorrhage (ICH); lacunar stroke (LACS); modified Rankin Scale (mRS); National Institute for Health Stroke Scale (NIHSS); non-stroke (N/S); partial anterior circulation stroke (PACS); posterior circulation stroke (POCS); transient ischaemic attack (TIA); total anterior circulation stroke (TACS).

Patients who ended up with a non-stroke diagnosis (*n* = 109) were a diverse group (diagnoses included migraine, subarachnoid haemorrhage and vasovagal events). Of these, 20 (18%) were untestable in some way. Only 12 patients (2%) of the full sample declined the cognitive assessment; three declined the full assessment and nine declined certain questions. Characteristics: 7 (58%) males, mean age of 74.3 (SD = 13.9), median NIHSS of 3 (IQR 2–5), diagnoses: 1 non-stroke, 3 TIAs, 3 PACS, 3 POCS and 2 LACS.

We looked at the completion of each individual question within our full cognitive assessment (Table S1). Clock-draw had the lowest completion rate (533/703 (76%)), whilst age had the highest (583/703 (83%)). For 25/58 (43%) patients in the partially untestable group, clock-draw was the only task that they did not attempt. The completion rate of each individual test is given in Table 2; the 4AT was the only test which could be scored in full for all patients.

In the univariate analyses: higher age, TACS, ICH, higher NIHSS, higher pre-morbid mRS and a previous diagnosis of dementia were associated with being untestable, whilst a lacunar stroke was associated with being testable (Table 4). In the first multivariable regression analysis (*n* = 680), independent associations with fully untestable status were: higher NIHSS score (OR: 1.18, 95% CI: 1.11–1.26), higher pre-morbid mRS (OR: 1.28, 95% CI: 1.02–1.60) and pre-stroke dementia (OR: 3.35, 95% CI: 1.53–7.32). A lacunar stroke classification was associated with being testable (OR: 0.19, 95% CI: 0.06–0.65). In the second analysis (where the partially untestable group was combined with the fully untestable), the above variables remained significant. In addition, the following associations were found for being untestable: older age (OR: 1.04, 95% CI: 1.02–1.06) and presence of ICH (OR: 3.44, 95% CI: 1.13–10.44); whilst a TIA classification was associated with being testable (OR: 0.45, 95% CI: 0.20–0.997) (Table 4).

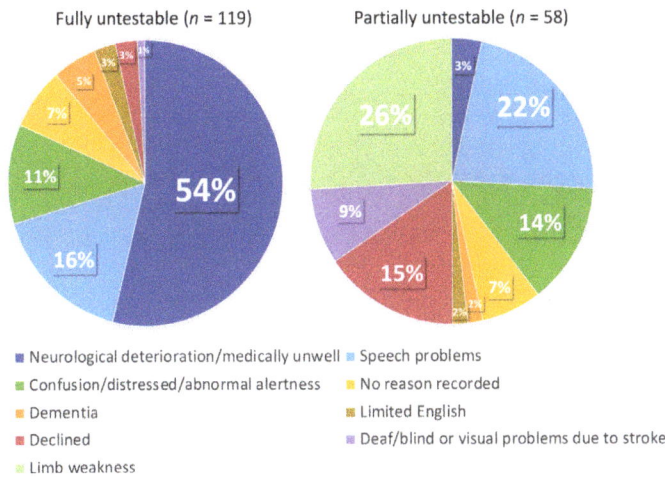

Figure 1. Reasons for fully/partially untestable.

Table 4. Feasibility associations.

Variables	Univariate for Fully Untestable	Multivariate (Partially Treated as Testable)	Multivariate (Partially Treated as Untestable)
	OR (95% CI)	OR (95% CI)	OR (95% CI)
Age (years)	**1.06 (1.04–1.08)**	1.02 (1.00–1.04)	**1.04 (1.02–1.06)**
Sex (male)	0.80 (0.54–1.18)	1.32 (0.77–2.26)	0.97 (0.62–1.51)
Stroke classification (non-stroke used as reference group):			
TACS	**23.08 (10.29–51.76)**	2.96 (0.98–8.93)	1.47 (0.50–4.34)
PACS	1.60 (0.80–3.22)	0.73 (0.32–1.65)	0.92 (0.46–1.83)
LACS	**0.28 (0.08–0.88)**	**0.19 (0.06–0.65)**	**0.26 (0.10–0.64)**
POCS	0.64 (0.25–1.62)	0.39 (0.14–1.12)	0.73 (0.33–1.61)
TIA	0.65 (0.28–1.50)	0.55 (0.21–1.40)	**0.45 (0.20–1.00 *)**
ICH	**2.96 (1.21–7.23)**	2.48 (0.72–8.59)	**3.44 (1.13–10.44)**
NIHSS	**1.30 (1.23–1.36)**	**1.18 (1.11–1.26)**	**1.23 (1.14–1.31)**
Pre-morbid mRS	**1.64 (1.41–1.91)**	**1.28 (1.02–1.60)**	**1.24 (1.03–1.50)**
Pre-stroke diagnosis of dementia	**6.01 (3.47–10.42)**	**3.35 (1.53–7.32)**	**2.74 (1.32–5.70)**
Previous stroke (IS, ICH) or TIA	0.96 (0.62–1.47)	0.82 (0.45–1.48)	0.91 (0.56–1.49)

* 0.997. Bold: significant associations. Abbreviations: intracerebral haemorrhage (ICH); ischaemic stroke (IS); lacunar stroke (LACS); modified Rankin Scale (mRS); National Institute for Health Stroke Scale (NIHSS); partial anterior circulation stroke (PACS); posterior circulation stroke (POCS); total anterior circulation stroke (TACS); transient ischemic attack (TIA).

4. Discussion

In an unselected sample of 703 patients admitted to our HASU, a quarter were classified as partially or fully untestable on brief cognitive screening tests. In those patients classified as partially untestable, the clock-draw was the most problematic, so tests including this item had the lowest completion rate. The 4AT was the only test which could be scored in full for all patients as it includes a score for being untestable. Factors associated with being fully untestable were previous diagnosis of dementia, higher pre-morbid mRS and higher NIHSS on admission, whilst a diagnosis of lacunar stroke was associated with being testable.

4.1. Research in Context

Our findings are generally in keeping with the limited literature on test feasibility. The associations of non-completion with stroke severity and dementia have face validity and the reasons given for a label of untestable were similar to those described in previous studies (for example limb weakness [5,11,16], aphasia [5,10,11], pre-morbid functional status [5] and reduced consciousness [11]), although reporting reasons for cognitive test non-completion in research is the exception rather than the norm. These findings highlight that non-completion is driven by both stroke specific and non-stroke related factors. Our finding that the clock-draw was the most problematic test is also in keeping with previous research findings for a stroke population; Lees et al. [16] found the lowest rates of completion on test items that required copying or drawing. Although tasks which assess visuospatial abilities, such as the clock-drawing test, can be challenging for stroke patients, they provide useful information on a key cognitive domain and can predict longer-term outcomes [32].

We decided to focus on the shortest cognitive tests available, in the hopes that they would be more practical for both the patient and clinician. Our results showed that the rates of completion for these short tests were similar to the completion rates for longer multi-domain cognitive tests previously studied (MoCA, MMSE). This should not be interpreted as meaning that the shortest tests are just as likely to be incomplete as more detailed tests. We did not include or directly compare longer tests with our short screens and our unselected population is not comparable with the patients tested in previous studies. There is a concern that shorter cognitive tests are inferior to longer, more detailed tests. Previous work has suggested that there is a trade-off between duration of administration and diagnostic accuracy [33] in the context of dementia. A focus on length of assessment alone (number of questions, administration time) is perhaps too simplistic, and test content is likely to be more important. For example, a long test could assess one area of cognition in depth yet neglect other domains.

4.2. Strengths and Weaknesses of the Research

A major strength of our study is that we had access to an unbiased, real-world sample, including patients who are often excluded from research (for example those with severe aphasia and dementia). While using clinical data have these benefits, we also have to acknowledge that due to the 'messy reality' of acute clinical practice, data are often missing. Our approach allowed us to retrospectively derive missing data from various sources including inpatient medical records, primary care data and consultation with the parent clinical team. Retrospective scoring can increase some inaccuracy, for example, calculating NIHSS based on the symptoms documented in medical case notes, rather than carrying it out directly with the patient.

There were some potentially interesting aspects of feasibility/applicability where we did not record data. We did not record the total number of patients who had limb weakness from their stroke and attempted the clock-draw using their weak or non-dominant hand (classed as testable). Data on this subgroup would be useful as many will lose points or score zero for poorly completed drawing tasks. We also did not record if an assessment had to be completed over two sessions or if any part of the assessment was interrupted.

Although we operationalised our concept of partially and fully untestable there is still subjectivity in the interpretation. It is essentially a judgement call by the clinician whether patients with aphasia, limb weakness and visual problems can complete a task (if the patient does not decline themselves). The same patient could therefore be classified differently purely based on who assessed them. This is particularly relevant in our study, where differing assessors performed the cognitive testing. This could be considered both a strength and weakness as it provides further real-world validity (some people might be better at encouraging patients to complete an assessment than others).

Finally, a limitation of determining feasibility of different questions and their resulting tests is the order in which the questions are asked. We acknowledge asking questions in the same order for each patient introduces some bias and is an issue because some patients will struggle to focus for longer periods of time or are easily fatigued.

4.3. Recommendations for Future Research and Practice

The strict administration and scoring criteria required for cognitive tests can be problematic for the stroke setting. Clinicians and researchers can therefore expect to encounter a number of stroke patients that will be untestable on certain tasks, or patients who are testable, but their stroke-related impairments result in a misleading test score. While in clinical practice an assessment can be put into context, in research it is more important that a-priori rules are set for dealing with incomplete tests. The importance of doing this is highlighted by the fact our analyses showed different results depending on how partially untestable patients were classified. Numerous approaches exist to deal with missing data [16], but to maximise the utility of the data collected, we recommend, where possible, that researchers make full use of incomplete participant data, rather than applying a complete-case analysis approach.

Tests which incorporate scoring for untestable patients, such as the 4AT, are helpful. Although the 4AT is primarily a delirium screen, the same approach could be applied to general cognitive tests. Guidance documents exist for scoring other stroke scales such as the NIHSS in patients who are comatose, confused, etc., so these types of resources could be made available for challenging cases in cognitive assessment.

Test completion rates are just one measure of feasibility. Feasibility covers a range of factors relating to the patient, assessor and the ward setting (Figure 2), so future research studies should include data addressing these other perspectives. To date, there has been little data published on the clinician's experience of cognitive assessment, environmental factors affecting assessment on the ward (noise, space, interruptions) and practical aspects, such as how assessors have misinterpreted administration/scoring instructions. With the increased use of computerised versions of cognitive tests in the future, feasibility issues from the assessor's side are likely to improve; for example, automatic scoring saves time and reduces scoring errors and subjectivity. Future research should also make use of routinely collected clinical data, such as that collected by the Sentinel Stroke National Audit Programme (SSNAP) and the Scottish stroke care audit in the United Kingdom. One could argue that any study using a researcher to administer a scale, rather than a clinical member of staff, is not truly addressing broader feasibility and implementation issues.

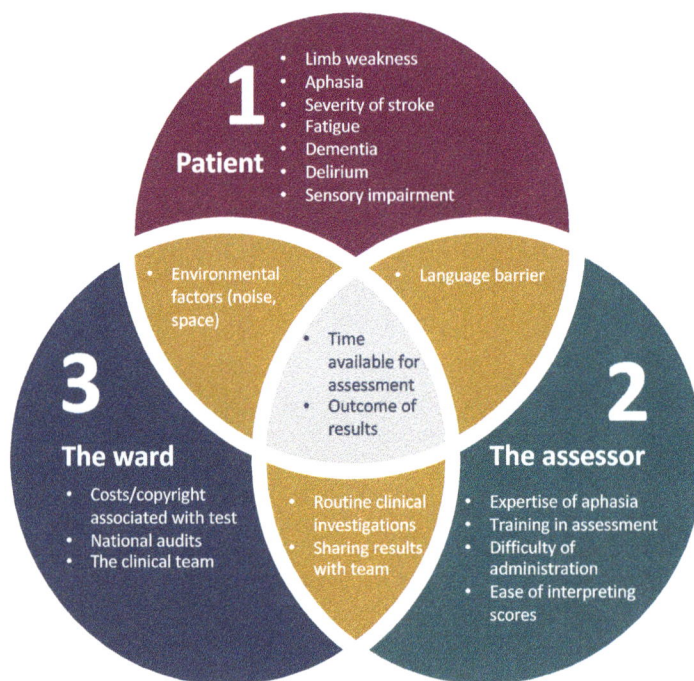

Figure 2. Factors affecting feasibility of cognitive assessment in acute stroke. Factors listed are illustrative but not exhaustive.

5. Conclusions

In a real-world sample, a quarter of patients in our HASU were classified as fully or partially untestable on brief cognitive screening tests. Clinicians and researchers should make a-priori plans on how to address incomplete assessments. Feasibility is a multi-faceted term, and factors from both clinician and patient point of view should be considered.

Supplementary Materials: The following are available online at http://www.mdpi.com/2075-4418/9/3/95/s1, Table S1: Questions attempted by the partially untestable group (*n* = 58).

Author Contributions: Conceptualisation, T.J.Q.; data collection, E.E., B.A.D., M.T.-R., R.C.S., G.C.; formal Analysis, E.E.; writing-original draft, E.E.; writing-reviewing & editing, all authors; supervision, T.J.Q.

Funding: This research was funded by the Stroke Association, grant number PPA 2015/01_CSO.

Conflicts of Interest: The authors declare no conflict of interest.

References

1. Quinn, T.J.; Elliott, E.; Langhorne, P. Cognitive and Mood Assessment Tools for Use in Stroke. *Stroke* **2018**, *49*, 483–490. [CrossRef] [PubMed]
2. Intercollegiate Stroke Working Party. *National Clinical Guideline for Stroke*, 5th ed.; Royal College of Physicians: London, UK, 2016.
3. Nasreddine, Z.S.; Phillips, N.A.; Bedirian, V.; Charbonneau, S.; Whitehead, V.; Collin, I.; Cummings, J.L.; Chertkow, H. The Montreal Cognitive Assessment, MoCA: A brief screening tool for mild cognitive impairment. *J. Am. Geriatr. Soc.* **2005**, *53*, 695–699. [CrossRef] [PubMed]
4. Folstein, M.F.; Folstein, S.E.; McHugh, P.R. "Mini-mental state". A practical method for grading the cognitive state of patients for the clinician. *J. Psychiatr Res.* **1975**, *12*, 189–198. [CrossRef]

5. Pasi, M.; Salvadori, E.; Poggesi, A.; Inzitari, D.; Pantoni, L. Factors predicting the Montreal cognitive assessment (MoCA) applicability and performances in a stroke unit. *J. Neurol* **2013**, *260*, 1518–1526. [CrossRef] [PubMed]

6. Benaim, C.; Barnay, J.L.; Wauquiez, G.; Bonnin-Koang, H.Y.; Anquetil, C.; Perennou, D.; Piscicelli, C.; Lucas-Pineau, B.; Muja, L.; le Stunff, E.; et al. The Cognitive Assessment scale for Stroke Patients (CASP) vs. MMSE and MoCA in non-aphasic hemispheric stroke patients. *Ann. Phys. Rehabil. Med.* **2015**, *58*, 78–85. [CrossRef] [PubMed]

7. van Zandvoort, M.J.E.; Kessels, R.P.C.; Nys, G.M.S.; de Haan, E.H.F.; Kappelle, L.J. Early neuropsychological evaluation in patients with ischaemic stroke provides valid information. *Clin. Neurol. Neurosurg.* **2005**, *107*, 385–392. [CrossRef]

8. Alderman, S.; Vahidy, F.; Bursaw, A.; Savitz, S. Abstract TP337: Feasibility of Cognitive Testing in Patients with Acute Ischemic Stroke. *Stroke* **2013**, *44*, ATP337. [CrossRef]

9. Collas, D. Detecting Cognitive Impairment in Acute Stroke Using the Oxford Cognitive Screen: Characteristics of Left and Right Hemisphere Strokes, with More Severe Impairment in AF Strokes (P1.190). *Neurology* **2016**, *86*, P1.190.

10. Horstmann, S.; Rizos, T.; Rauch, G.; Arden, C.; Veltkamp, R. Feasibility of the Montreal Cognitive Assessment in acute stroke patients. *Eur. J. Neurol.* **2014**, *21*, 1387–1393. [CrossRef]

11. Pendlebury, S.T.; Klaus, S.P.; Thomson, R.J.; Mehta, Z.; Wharton, R.M.; Rothwell, P.M. Methodological Factors in Determining Risk of Dementia After Transient Ischemic Attack and Stroke: (III) Applicability of Cognitive Tests. *Stroke* **2015**, *46*, 3067–3073. [CrossRef]

12. Barnay, J.L.; Wauquiez, G.; Bonnin-Koang, H.Y.; Anquetil, C.; Perennou, D.; Piscicelli, C.; Lucas-Pineau, B.; Muja, L.; le Stunff, E.; de Boissezon, X.; et al. Feasibility of the cognitive assessment scale for stroke patients (CASP) vs. MMSE and MoCA in aphasic left hemispheric stroke patients. *Ann. Phys. Rehabil. Med.* **2014**, *57*, 422–435. [CrossRef]

13. Cumming, T.B.; Bernhardt, J.; Linden, T. The montreal cognitive assessment: Short cognitive evaluation in a large stroke trial. *Stroke* **2011**, *42*, 2642–2644. [CrossRef]

14. Kwa, V.I.H.; Limburg, M.; Voogel, A.J.; Teunisse, S.; Derix, M.M.A.; Hijdra, A. Feasibility of cognitive screening of patients with ischaemic stroke using the CAMCOG A hospital-based study. *J. Neurol.* **1996**, *243*, 405–409. [CrossRef]

15. Mancuso, M.; Demeyere, N.; Abbruzzese, L.; Damora, A.; Varalta, V.; Pirrotta, F.; Antonucci, G.; Matano, A.; Caputo, M.; Caruso, M.G.; et al. Using the Oxford Cognitive Screen to Detect Cognitive Impairment in Stroke Patients: A Comparison with the Mini-Mental State Examination. *Front. Neurol.* **2018**, *9*, 101. [CrossRef]

16. Lees, R.A.; Hendry Ba, K.; Broomfield, N.; Stott, D.; Larner, A.J.; Quinn, T.J. Cognitive assessment in stroke: Feasibility and test properties using differing approaches to scoring of incomplete items. *Int. J. Geriatr. Psychiatry* **2017**, *32*, 1072–1078. [CrossRef]

17. Pendlebury, S.T.; Chen, P.J.; Bull, L.; Silver, L.; Mehta, Z.; Rothwell, P.M. Methodological factors in determining rates of dementia in transient ischemic attack and stroke: (I) impact of baseline selection bias. *Stroke* **2015**, *46*, 641–646. [CrossRef]

18. Demeyere, N.; Riddoch, M.J.; Slavkova, E.D.; Bickerton, W.L.; Humphreys, G.W. The Oxford Cognitive Screen (OCS): Validation of a stroke-specific short cognitive screening tool. *Psychol. Assess.* **2015**, *27*, 883–894. [CrossRef]

19. Bennett, D.A.; Brayne, C.; Feigin, V.L.; Barker-Collo, S.; Brainin, M.; Davis, D.; Gallo, V.; Jette, N.; Karch, A.; Kurtzke, J.F.; et al. Development of the standards of reporting of neurological disorders (STROND) checklist: A guideline for the reporting of incidence and prevalence studies in neuroepidemiology. *Eur. J. Epidemiol.* **2015**, *30*, 569–576. [CrossRef]

20. Brott, T.; Adams, H.P., Jr.; Olinger, C.P.; Marler, J.R.; Barsan, W.G.; Biller, J.; Spilker, J.; Holleran, R.; Eberle, R.; Hertzberg, V.; et al. Measurements of acute cerebral infarction: A clinical examination scale. *Stroke* **1989**, *20*, 864–870. [CrossRef]

21. Rankin, J. Cerebral vascular accidents in patients over the age of 60. I. General considerations. *Scott. Med. J.* **1957**, *2*, 127–136. [CrossRef]

22. van Swieten, J.C.; Koudstaal, P.J.; Visser, M.C.; Schouten, H.J.; van Gijn, J. Interobserver agreement for the assessment of handicap in stroke patients. *Stroke* **1988**, *19*, 604–607. [CrossRef]

23. Fearon, P.; McArthur, K.S.; Garrity, K.; Graham, L.J.; McGroarty, G.; Vincent, S.; Quinn, T.J. Prestroke modified rankin stroke scale has moderate interobserver reliability and validity in an acute stroke setting. *Stroke* **2012**, *43*, 3184–3188. [CrossRef]

24. Hodkinson, H.M. Evaluation of a mental test score for assessment of mental impairment in the elderly. *Age Ageing* **1972**, *1*, 233–238. [CrossRef]

25. Swain, D.G.; Nightingale, P.G. Evaluation of a shortened version of the Abbreviated Mental Test in a series of elderly patients. *Clin. Rehabil.* **1997**, *11*, 243–248. [CrossRef]

26. Brodaty, H.; Pond, D.; Kemp, N.M.; Luscombe, G.; Harding, L.; Berman, K.; Huppert, F.A. The GPCOG: A new screening test for dementia designed for general practice. *J. Am. Geriatr. Soc.* **2002**, *50*, 530–534. [CrossRef]

27. Borson, S.; Scanlan, J.M.; Chen, P.; Ganguli, M. The Mini-Cog as a screen for dementia: Validation in a population-based sample. *J. Am. Geriatr. Soc.* **2003**, *51*, 1451–1454. [CrossRef]

28. Brooke, P.; Bullock, R. Validation of a 6 item cognitive impairment test with a view to primary care usage. *Int. J. Geriatr. Psychiatry* **1999**, *14*, 936–940. [CrossRef]

29. Hachinski, V.; Iadecola, C.; Petersen, R.C.; Breteler, M.M.; Nyenhuis, D.L.; Black, S.E.; Powers, W.J.; DeCarli, C.; Merino, J.G.; Kalaria, R.N.; et al. National Institute of Neurological Disorders and Stroke-Canadian Stroke Network vascular cognitive impairment harmonization standards. *Stroke* **2006**, *37*, 2220–2241. [CrossRef]

30. Panenková, E.; Kopecek, M.; Lukavsky, J. Item analysis and possibility to abbreviate the Montreal Cognitive Assessment. *Ceska Slov. Psychiatr.* **2016**, *112*, 63–69.

31. Ismail, Z.; Rajji, T.K.; Shulman, K.I. Brief cognitive screening instruments: An update. *Int. J. Geriatr. Psychiatry* **2010**, *25*, 111–120. [CrossRef]

32. Champod, A.S.; Gubitz, G.J.; Phillips, S.J.; Christian, C.; Reidy, Y.; Radu, L.M.; Darvesh, S.; Reid, J.M.; Kintzel, F.; Eskes, G.A. Clock Drawing Test in acute stroke and its relationship with long-term functional and cognitive outcomes. *Clin. Neuropsychol.* **2019**, *33*, 817–830. [CrossRef] [PubMed]

33. Larner, A.J. Speed versus accuracy in cognitive assessment when using CSIs. *Prog. Neurol. Psychiatry* **2015**, *19*, 21–24. [CrossRef]

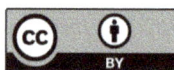

diagnostics

MDPI

Review

Thirty-Five Years of Computerized Cognitive Assessment of Aging—Where Are We Now?

Avital Sternin [1,*], Alistair Burns [2] and Adrian M. Owen [1,3]

[1] Brain and Mind Institute, Department of Psychology, University of Western Ontario, London, ON N6A 3K7, Canada
[2] Division of Neuroscience & Experimental Psychology, Manchester Institute for Collaborative Research on Ageing, School of Social Sciences, University of Manchester, Manchester M13 9PL, UK
[3] Department of Physiology and Pharmacology, University of Western Ontario, London, ON N6A 3K7, Canada
* Correspondence: avital.sternin@uwo.ca

Received: 30 August 2019; Accepted: 3 September 2019; Published: 6 September 2019

Abstract: Over the past 35 years, the proliferation of technology and the advent of the internet have resulted in many reliable and easy to administer batteries for assessing cognitive function. These approaches have great potential for affecting how the health care system monitors and screens for cognitive changes in the aging population. Here, we review these new technologies with a specific emphasis on what they offer over and above traditional 'paper-and-pencil' approaches to assessing cognitive function. Key advantages include fully automated administration and scoring, the interpretation of individual scores within the context of thousands of normative data points, the inclusion of 'meaningful change' and 'validity' indices based on these large norms, more efficient testing, increased sensitivity, and the possibility of characterising cognition in samples drawn from the general population that may contain hundreds of thousands of test scores. The relationship between these new computerized platforms and existing (and commonly used) paper-and-pencil tests is explored, with a particular emphasis on why computerized tests are particularly advantageous for assessing the cognitive changes associated with aging.

Keywords: computerized cognitive assessment; aging; dementia; memory; executive function

---

1. Introduction

Cognitive assessment has been of interest to psychology, cognitive neuroscience, and general medicine for more than 150 years. In the earliest reports, such as the widely-discussed case of Phineas Gage [1], cognitive 'assessment' was based solely on observation and subjective reports of the behavioural changes that followed a serendipitous brain injury. By the early 20th century, there had been several attempts to standardize cognitive assessments by individuals such as James Cattell [2] and Alfred Binet [3], although these were few and far between, often based on subsets of cognitive processes, and designed with specific populations in mind (e.g., children). It was not until the 1950s, 60s and 70s that the field of cognitive assessment exploded, and dozens of batteries of tests were developed, 'normed', and made widely available for general use (e.g., the Wechsler Adult Intelligence Scale [4], the Wechsler Memory Scale [5], the Stroop task [6,7]).

In the 1980s, a shift in emphasis occurred, as portable computers became more accessible and existing 'paper and pencil' cognitive assessments began to be digitized. Finally, by the turn of the century, the emergence of the world wide web made 'internet based' testing a reality, resulting in the creation of more reliable and efficient tests that could be taken from anywhere in the world. In parallel with the development of computerized tests for cognitive assessment, computerized brain-training games have also become popular (e.g., Lumosity). In this paper, we will only be discussing batteries designed for assessment (rather than 'training') purposes. Despite the proliferation of both laboratory-based and internet-based computerized cognitive assessment platforms and the many advantages they offer, these systems are still not as widely used as many of the classic paper-and-pencil batteries, particularly in older adult populations. For example, a PsychInfo search for peer-reviewed journal articles published in the 10 years between 1 July 2009 and 1 July 2019 that used the Wechsler Adult Intelligence Scale [4] and the Mini-Mental State Examination [8] in participants over the age of 65 returned 983 and 2224 studies, respectively. By comparison, when the same parameters were used to search for 'computerized cognitive assessment' only 364 results were returned.

The goal of this paper is to provide an overview of how both laboratory-based and internet-based cognitive assessments have evolved since the 1980s when computerized approaches were first introduced to the present day when they routinely make use of small, ultra-portable technologies such as cell phones and tablets (e.g., iPads). We will focus our discussion on how these assessments are being applied to detect and track dementia. Key differences between these new computerized platforms and existing (and commonly used) paper-and-pencil tests will be discussed, with a particular emphasis on why computerized tests are particularly advantageous for assessing the cognitive changes associated with aging.

2. Computerized Cognitive Assessment—Historically

The computerization of cognitive assessment tools began in the 1980s with the development of personal computers. Although initial digitization efforts mainly focused on the straight conversion of paper-and-pencil tests to computerized formats, new methods of assessment soon began to be developed that capitalized on emerging technologies (such as touchscreens, response pads, computer mice, etc.). These new methods, when used alongside computers to collect data, led to the creation of tests that were more efficient at assessing an individual's abilities than their paper-and-pencil equivalents. For example, computerized tests are able to measure response latencies with millisecond accuracy and record and report on many aspects of performance simultaneously. Computers can calculate scores and modify test difficulty on the fly, as well as automate instructions, practice questions, and administration of the tests across large groups of people—something that is not so easy for a human test administrator to accomplish. Moreover, because test difficulty can be adjusted on-the-fly, assessments can be shorter and therefore less frustrating, or exhausting, for impaired individuals. In addition, predefined criteria can dictate the maximum number of successes or failures that each individual is exposed to, such that the subjective experience of being tested is equivalent across participants. The reporting of scores also becomes easier and more accurate because their interpretation can be made entirely objectively based on calculated statistics using information gleaned from large normative datasets.

Some of these advantages lead to greater test sensitivity [9] and as such, computerized cognitive assessments are valuable for investigating changes that may not be detected using conventional methods. This makes them ideal for assessing and following subtle cognitive changes in aging over the long term and increases the possibility that emerging mild cognitive impairments will be detected as early as possible [10].

An early example of a set of computerized cognitive tests was the Cambridge Neuropsychological Test Automated Battery (CANTAB). CANTAB was originally designed for the neuropsychological assessment of neurodegenerative diseases and was the first touch-screen based, comprehensive, computerized cognitive battery. CANTAB was standardized in nearly 800 older adult participants [11], and early studies indicated that specific tests, or combinations of tests, were sensitive to deficits and progressive decline in both Alzheimer's disease and Parkinson's disease [12–16]. Specific tests from the CANTAB battery also appear to be able to predict the development of dementia in preclinical populations, while also differentiating between different disorders such as Alzheimer's disease and Frontotemporal dementia [10,17,18]. This early example of a computerized neuropsychological battery paved the way for others, designed to assess similar, or different, types of cognitive function and dysfunction (e.g., Cambridge Brain Sciences [19], Automatic Neuropsychological Assessment

Metrics [20], Computerized Neuropsychological Test Battery [21], Touch Panel-Type Dementia Assessment Scale [22]).

Although the broad body of literature that has accumulated over the last 35 years indicates that computerized tests are adept at detecting and monitoring cognitive decline in neurodegenerative disorders, little consensus exists about which are the most effective and suitable for this task. Two recent reviews described 17 such batteries as being suitable for use in aging populations (see [23,24] for tables illustrating these batteries in detail). The consensus across both reviews was that, although broadly valid for testing aging populations, many of these batteries had serious shortcomings. For example, many batteries relied on normative data from small samples sizes or samples that lacked data specific to older adults. Ultimately, both reviews suggested that how useful any given battery was must be assessed on a case-by-case basis and that no one test, or battery of tests, could be singled out as being the most reliable for screening and monitoring cognitive impairment in the elderly. Without doubt, this general lack of consensus about computerized cognitive tests has contributed to their slow adoption into health care systems. Clinicians are rightly hesitant to adopt any new platform for screening or monitoring patients when normative population data are lacking [25], and this issue needs to be urgently resolved. The obvious way to accomplish this is to greatly increase the number of participants who have completed any given computerized test or battery, and generate norms based on these large databases that can be used to assess the performance of groups or individuals with known, or suspected, clinical disorders. For practical and economic reasons, this is not feasible when assessments need to be taken by a trained administrator in a laboratory testing environment. However, with the advent of the internet, mass 'self-administration' of computerized cognitive tests has become a reality, opening up many new and transformative opportunities in this domain.

3. Cognitive Assessment in the Internet Age

The internet and the proliferation of portable computers into every aspect of our lives (e.g., phones, TVs, tablets), has created many new opportunities, and challenges, for computerized cognitive assessment. For example, by making cognitive assessments available online, a much larger number of participants can be reached than would be possible when the tests are administered on paper and/or in a laboratory setting. With increasing numbers, demographic variables such as age, geographical location and socioeconomic status can also be fed into each assessment, and on-the-fly comparisons with large normative databases can be used to provide 'personalized' results that take these factors into account.

One example of such an online tool is the Cambridge Brain Sciences (CBS) platform. The tests in this battery are largely based on well validated neuropsychological tasks but have been adapted and designed to capitalize on the numerous advantages that internet and computer-based testing can offer. The CBS battery has been used to conduct several large-scale population-based studies involving tens of thousands of participants from all over the world [19,26], as well as more than 300 bespoke scientific studies (e.g., [27–29]). As testament to the 'power of the internet', in total, more than 8 million tests have been taken, and normative data from 75,000 healthy participants are available, including approximately 5000 adults over the age of 65.

Having access to such a large number of datapoints also makes it possible to investigate how demographic factors affect cognition in a way and on a scale that was never before feasible, shedding new light on the interplay between biology and environmental factors and their effects on cognitive function. For example, in one recent study of 45,000 individuals, the CBS battery was used to examine the influence of factors like gender differences, anxiety, depression, substance abuse, and socio-economic status on cognitive function, as well as how they interact during the aging process to uniquely affect different aspects of performance [30].

Other computerized assessment batteries that have been used in older adult populations include the Automatic Neuropsychological Assessment Metrics [20], Computerized Neuropsychological Test Battery [21], and the Touch Panel-Type Dementia Assessment Scale [22]. Each of these batteries consists of a series of tests designed to measure various aspects of cognitive functioning such as processing speed, memory retention, and working memory using tasks based on command following, object recognition, logical reasoning, mathematical processing, and symbol-digit coding.

3.1. Meaningful Change

When normative databases include tens of thousands of participants, it becomes possible to compute indices that are simply not possible with smaller (e.g., lab-based) data samples. Estimates of 'meaningful' or 'reliable' change are one such example that has particular relevance for monitoring cognitive decline or improvement on an individual basis. Estimates of meaningful or reliable change compare the difference in an individual's performance on a task between two time points (e.g., between a patient's current assessment results and previous baseline results) to the variability in repeated measurements that would occur in the absence of a meaningful change. The latter is estimated from a sample of healthy control subjects, and the larger that sample is, the better. Gathering data from a large number of individuals via online testing allows for a database of thousands of normative data points [19,31]. The meaningful change index used by the CBS platform, for example, uses the test-retest reliability and the standard deviation of scores (measured in the control sample) of each task to describe the range of possible differences that could occur with repeated task completion. If an individual's change in performance from one time point to another is much larger than expected by chance (i.e., larger than the fluctuations seen in the control sample), then one can conclude that there was a meaningful change. This may be crucial for evaluating a single aging patient and deciding whether or not a change in performance from one assessment to the next is 'meaningful' or simply a reflection of the day to day fluctuations that are characteristic of healthy cognitive functioning. The above method of calculating a meaningful change score is one example of how computerized cognitive testing can be used to monitor cognitive changes over time. Other methods that, for example, investigate the longitudinal measurement invariance can also be used [32,33] to determine whether the scores from a single metric collected over time are stable or changing in a meaningful way.

The increased size of the normative database to which individual scores are compared is one way in which modern internet-based assessment tools are able to address an issue raised by Zygouris and Tsolaki [24]; that is, physicians rarely have time to wade through the complicated data output of computerized testing batteries to interpret their meaning. When the meaning of test results can be determined through automated statistical algorithms that interrogate a large normative database, the task of interpreting test results is offloaded to the battery itself (something that is clearly not possible with traditional pencil-and-paper methods). When a meaningful change is detected, caregivers or health care providers can be alerted 'automatically' so that more in-depth testing can be initiated to assess the individual's cognitive status. This has relevance in home care, assisted living facilities, and in hospital settings for reducing the administrative burden of monitoring cognitive changes, while also increasing the sensitivity of testing to catch important changes early enough to be appropriately addressed. This in turn, increases the likelihood that physicians will be amenable to adopting these methods for monitoring and screening aging individuals because the logistic and economic overheads are low. In addition, the immediate delivery, objectivity, and interpretation of scores makes them straightforward for non-experts to understand and increases the probability that these methods will be adopted into the broader health care system because any health care provider or family member can, in principle, monitor an aging patient's cognitive changes over time, the effect of drugs, or even cognitive changes post-surgically [34].

3.2. Validity of At-Home Testing

As we have implied above, one of the main advantages of internet-based testing is that it can be conducted at home (or theoretically, anywhere), as long as a computer with an internet connection is available. One of the obvious questions, however, is its validity in comparison to in-lab testing. To assess this question, we had 19 healthy young adult control participants complete the full CBS battery (12 tests) both while unsupervised at home and while supervised in the laboratory (test order was counterbalanced across participants). The mean standardized scores for each of the tests showed no significant effect of at home versus in laboratory testing ($F = 1.71$, $p = 0.2$) and the tasks showed reliable correlations within participants across the two testing environments ($p < 0.05$) (See Figure 1A). A follow-up study explored whether the stability in scores across testing environments was applicable to patient groups as well as healthy controls. A total of 27 participants with Parkinson's disease were assessed on 4 of the 12 CBS tests at home and in-lab as well as tests of simple and choice reaction time similar to the ones included in the CANTAB battery (the order of tasks was counterbalanced across participants). Again, there was no significant effect of at home versus in-lab testing ($p > 0.1$), and the tasks showed reliable correlations across the two testing environments ($p < 0.05$) (See Figure 1B). Moreover, the results of the simple and choice reaction time tasks demonstrated that response time measures could be collected accurately over the internet, regardless of the testing platform used. Together, the results of these two studies indicate that computerized tests taken unsupervised at home produce results no different than those taken in a laboratory, both in healthy controls and in a patient population.

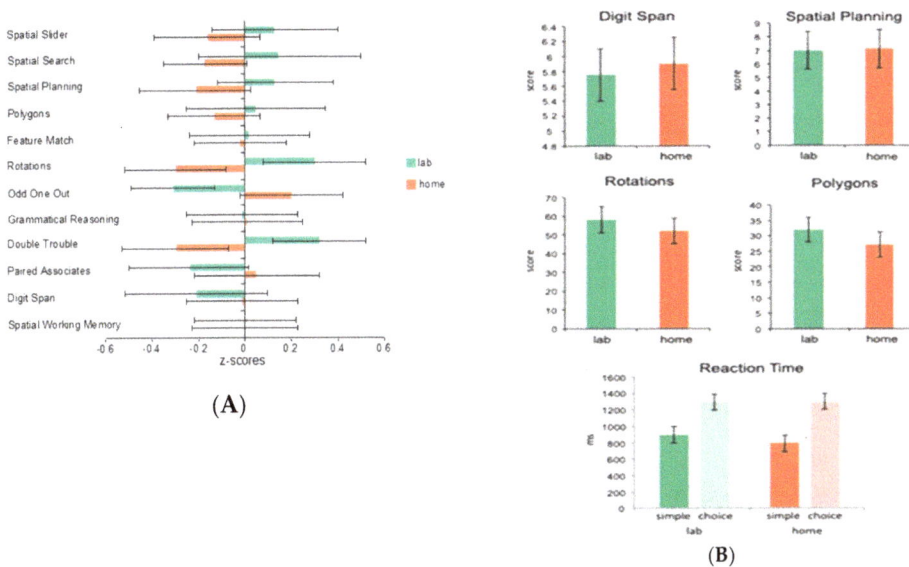

Figure 1. (**A**) average standardized scores on the 12 Cambridge Brain Sciences (CBS) tasks taken at home and in the lab by 19 healthy young adult controls. The results showed no significant effect of at home versus in laboratory testing ($F = 1.71$, $p = 0.2$); (**B**) average raw scores on 4 CBS tasks as well as simple and choice reaction time tasks taken at home and in the lab by 27 patients with Parkinson's Disease. Again, there was no significant effect of at home versus in-lab testing ($p > 0.1$) and the tasks showed reliable correlations across the two testing environments ($p < 0.05$).

In a third recently published study examining the relationship between unsupervised cognitive testing 'at home' and supervised lab-based assessment, the performance of more than 100 participants was compared on three of the CBS tests, Digit Span, Spatial Span and Token Search [35] There were no significant differences in performance between those participants who completed the tests online via Amazon's MTurk platform and those who completed the testing supervised within the laboratory (Figure 2). In the case of the Token Search test, this was even true after extensive training on the task over several weeks [35].

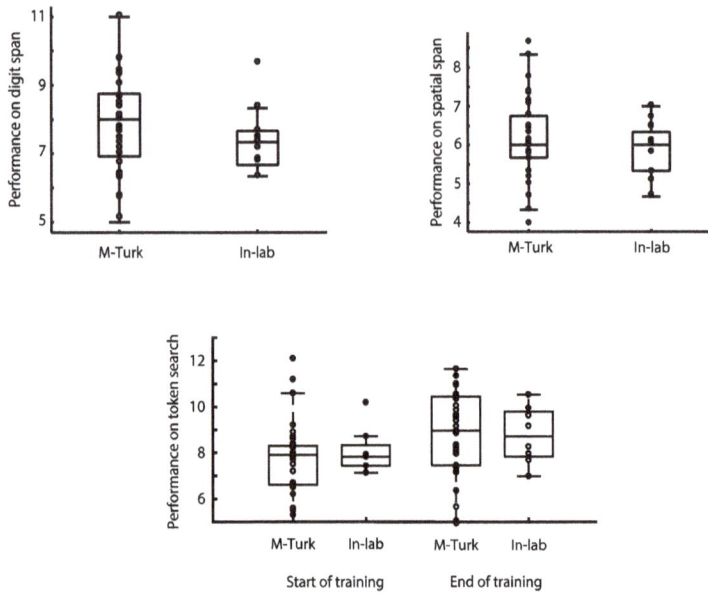

Figure 2. Average scores on 3 CBS tasks (Digit Span, Spatial Span and Token Search), taken at home and in the lab by more than 100 young adult controls. The results showed no significant effect of at home versus in laboratory testing [35]. In the case of Token Search (lower panel), the overlap in performance for participants tested at home using Amazon's MTurk and those tested in the laboratory persisted even after several weeks of intensive training on the task [35].

Another advantage of internet-based testing and large-scale normative databases is that it is relatively straightforward to calculate indicators of 'validity' on-the-fly which can then be used to 'flag' when testing has not been completed properly, or according to the instructions. By analyzing thousands of data points, a set of parameters can be defined that must be met for a score on a test to be considered valid. Including a simple and easy-to-read marker on a score report that conveys whether performance on a task is within reasonable bounds increases the usability and confidence in the test by health care providers.

Finally, there are other mechanisms that can be used to ensure reliable data are collected when tasks are self-administered at home in online settings. For example, interactive learning tutorials can guide participants through practice trials and objectively determine when an individual has understood task instructions before beginning a testing session. Such practice trials increase the validity of the tests, particularly when they are taken for the first time.

4. Online Testing vs. Existing Alternatives

The ability to quickly and accurately assess changes in cognitive functioning on a regular basis has implications for quality of life, level of independence, and degree of care in the aging adult population. Currently, assessments like the Mini-Mental Status Exam (MMSE) [8] and the Montreal Cognitive Assessment (MoCA) [36] are used by health care providers to monitor cognitive changes and screen for deficits. Although these tests are useful because they are short and easy to administer, there are some downsides to using these paper-and-pencil based methods of assessment. For example, they are not adaptive to an individual's ability level, which can lead to frustration in patients with deficits or unnecessary redundancy in individuals who are clearly completely unimpaired. In addition, the questions are not randomly generated with each administration (so opportunities for retesting are reduced). Third, these tests must be administered by a trained individual, which introduces testing bias and takes time and resources away from other health care duties. Fourth, rather than detecting fine grained changes in cognition, these paper-pencil tests assign patients to very broad categories (impaired or unimpaired)—binary classification of this sort is highly susceptible to error through day to day fluctuations in normal cognitive functioning. Finally, the cutoff scores used in these tests may not be appropriate for aging populations [37–39] and result in larger numbers of patients being labeled as 'impaired' than perhaps is necessary.

Several recent studies have investigated whether short computerized assessments can effectively monitor cognitive changes over time and better differentiate between older adult populations with differing abilities than the most widely used paper-and-pencil alternatives. When 45 older adults recruited from a geriatric psychiatry outpatient clinic were tested on five computerized tests from the CBS battery, results showed that some of these tests provided more information about each individual's cognitive abilities than the standard MoCA when administered on its own [40]. The addition of scores from just two of the computerized tests (total testing time of 6 min) to a MoCA, better sorted participants into impaired or unimpaired categories. Specifically, 81% of those patients who were classified as being borderline (between 'impaired' and 'not impaired') based on their MoCA scores alone were reclassified as one or the other when scores from two computerized tests were introduced. Additionally, this study demonstrated that some computerized tests provide more information than others when used in this context. That is to say, two of the five tests employed were not at all useful in classifying borderline patients and the fifth test was too difficult for the older adults to understand and complete.

To follow-up this study, we recently investigated whether other tests in the CBS battery, beyond the five used by Brenkel et al. [40], could provide more information about older adults' cognitive abilities, as well as whether traditional tests like the MoCA or the MMSE could be replaced entirely by an online computerized assessment battery.

A total of 52 older adults (average age = 81 years, 62–97 years) were asked to complete the 12 online tests from the CBS battery in random order. Each task was presented on a touchscreen tablet computer and was preceded by instructions and practice trials. Afterwards, the MoCA (version 7.1 English) and MMSE were administered in interview format, always by the same person (AS). Possibly because of the location of the retirement homes from which participants were recruited, the sample was highly educated. All but one earned high school diplomas, 24 earned postsecondary degrees, and 16 earned postgraduate degrees. Two participants did not complete all 12 tasks due to fatigue and loss of interest; thus 50 participants' scores were analysed. MoCA scores ranged from 12–30 (mean = 24.6) and MMSE scores ranged from 16–30 (mean = 27.7; see Supplementary Figure S1).

Participant scores were split into three categories based on the results of the MoCA test (See Figure 3): unimpaired (n = 25; MoCA score ≥ 26), borderline cognitive impairment (n = 14; MoCA score 23–25), and impaired (n = 12; MoCA score ≤ 22), based on thresholds from previous literature (e.g., [36–38]). Each participant in the borderline MoCA group was then reclassified to either the impaired or unimpaired groups based on their CBS test scores. A ceiling effect precluded such an analysis for the MMSE results.

Using the MoCA score alone, 72% of participants were classified as impaired or unimpaired. The addition of a single CBS task (Spatial Planning) improved this classification to 92% of the participants. This was not simply because Spatial Planning was the most difficult test, as the equally difficult Spatial Span test left 5 participants in the borderline group. Test difficulty was determined from an unrelated study with scores from 327 participants age 71–80 (see Supplementary Figure S2).

A second analysis using a step-wise multiple regression indicated that MoCA scores were best predicted by two additional CBS tests: Odd One Out and Feature Match (R^2 = 0.65). Age did not significantly predict any variance over and above these tests. Alone, age predicted 22% of the variance in MoCA scores (R^2 = 0.22). Another step-wise multiple regression showed that MMSE scores were best predicted by Feature Match and Grammatical Reasoning (R^2 = 0.38). Again, age did not explain a significant amount of variance over and above the task scores. Alone, age predicted 8% ($R^2 = 0.08$) of the variance in MMSE scores.

A third regression showed that level of education did not explain a significant amount of variance in MMSE or MoCA scores, although this may be due to overall high educational levels and the ceiling effect seen in MMSE scores (see Supplementary Figure S1).

Scores on the three CBS tasks identified in the two analyses (Feature Match, Odd One Out, Spatial Planning) were then combined to create a composite score. The composite score was highly correlated with MoCA scores and was better than the MoCA alone at differentiating impaired from unimpaired participants (84% versus 72% for the MoCA on its own; see Figure 3).

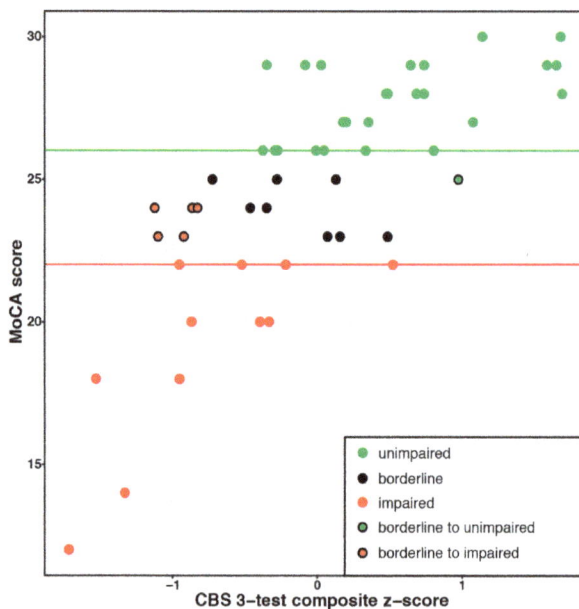

Figure 3. The CBS composite score was highly correlated with Montreal Cognitive Assessment (MoCA) scores and better differentiated impaired and unimpaired individuals. The border colour of each datapoint indicates the categorization of individuals based on MoCA scores alone. The fill colour indicates to which group borderline participants are categorized when the composite score of 3 CBS tests is used.

The results discussed above illustrate the potential that short computerized tests have as screening tools for efficiently monitoring cognitive changes over time. This study also suggests that minimal computer literacy is required when using a touchscreen tablet as technical limitations did not preclude individuals from participating. Another potential use for computerized testing is as a replacement for, or supplement to, neuropsychological assessments that are used for the diagnosis of various brain disorders. In one recent foray into this area, the relationship between a 30 min computerized testing battery and a standard 2–3 h neuropsychological assessment [41] was explored in 134 healthy adults (mean age was 47 years). Although the computerized testing battery could not account for significant variance in the assessments of verbal abilities (e.g., WASI Vocabulary subtest, Word List Generation), it did account for 61% of the variance in the remainder of the traditional neuropsychological battery. The results confirmed that a 30 min internet-based assessment of attention, memory, and executive functioning was comparable to a standard 2–3 h neuropsychological test battery and may even have some diagnostic capabilities.

In the sections above, we have sought to illustrate our arguments with just a few examples of how cognitive changes in older adults can be effectively monitored using self-administered, internet-based computerized testing batteries. Although further validation is required in some cases, there is already good reason to believe that a shift towards internet-based computerized cognitive testing in health care may be warranted.

5. Neural Validation

A key aspect to cognitive assessment is validating the areas of the brain that are involved in the cognitive functions in question. This has long been the domain of neuropsychologists who use results from neurally validated assessments to triangulate brain function from behavioural assessment results. Historically, cognitive assessments were validated using brain lesion studies, but the rise of imaging technologies has made the neural validation of newly developed cognitive assessments accessible and easier to complete.

Coincidentally, the computerization of cognitive assessments has grown alongside this increase in the availability of imaging tools. These parallel timelines have resulted in many examples of computerized cognitive tasks that have been validated from the get-go with neural information gleaned from neuroimaging studies [19,42]. Importantly, however, these imaging studies have underscored the fact that there is rarely a one-to-one mapping between cognitive functions and the brain areas, or networks, that underpin them. One approach to this issue is to examine the complex statistical relationships between performance on any one cognitive task (or group of tasks) and changes in brain activity to reveal how one is related to the other. In order to do this most effectively, large amounts of data need to be included because of the natural variance in cognitive performance (and brain activity) across tests and across individuals. In the age of computerized internet testing and so-called 'big data', this problem becomes much easier to solve. Thus, the sheer amount of data that can be collected allows statistical tests to be performed that were simply not possible when data were collected by hand. For example, Hampshire et al. [19] collected data on the 12 CBS tasks from 45,000 participants. These data were then subjected to a factor analysis, and 3 discrete factors relating to overall cognitive performance were identified. Each one of these factors represents an independent cognitive function that is best described by a combination of performance on multiple tests, something that no single test can assess, and were labeled as encapsulating aspects of short-term memory, reasoning, and verbal abilities, respectively. This technique allows an individual's performance to be compared to a very large normative database in terms of these descriptive factors rather than performance on a single test.

As an example of how this might be applied to a question related directly to aging, Wild et al. [31] recently used this same approach to investigate how sleeping patterns affect cognitive function across the lifespan in a global sample of more than 10,000 people. Using the same analysis of factor structure employed previously by Hampshire et al. [19], the results showed that the relationship between sleep and short-term memory, reasoning and verbal factors was invariant with respect to age, overturning the widely-held notion that the optimal amount of sleep is different in older age groups. Indeed, sleep-related impairments in these three aspects of cognition were shown to affect all ages equally, despite the fact that, as expected, older people tended to sleep less [31]. Put simply, the amount of sleep that resulted in optimal cognitive performance (7–8 h), and the impact of deviating from this amount, was the same for everyone—regardless of age. Somewhat counter-intuitively, this implies that older adults who slept more or less than the optimal amount were impacted no more than younger adults who had non-optimal sleep. If sleep is especially important for staving off dementia and age-related cognitive decline [43], then one might predict that a lack of sleep (or too much sleep) would be associated with more pronounced cognitive impairment in the elderly than in younger adults. Nonetheless, given that 7–8 h of sleep was associated with optimal cognition for all ages and that increasing age was associated with less sleep, the results suggest that older populations in general would likely benefit from more sleep.

Additionally, the neural networks responsible for cognitive factors that are derived from analysing data from multiple tests across large samples of participants can be assessed. For example, Hampshire et al. [19] described the neural correlates of each factor in a group of 16 healthy young participants who completed the testing battery in an fMRI scanner. The short-term memory factor was related to activation in the insula/frontal operculum, the superior frontal sulcus, and the ventral portion of the anterior cingulate cortex and pre-supplementary motor areas. The reasoning factor was related to activation in the inferior frontal sulcus, the inferior parietal cortex, and the dorsal portion of the anterior cingulate and pre-supplementary motor areas. The verbal factor was related to activation in the left inferior frontal gyrus and the bilateral temporal lobes. These data indicate that identifying the neural correlates of cognitive functions is possible with a very large database of participants allowing for complex statistical tests to be performed to interrogate their complex inter-relationships. Computerized assessments are particularly suited to the task of collecting thousands of datapoints and combined with imaging data can provide valuable insights into how a brain injury or neural degeneration as a result of aging affects the brain networks responsible for complex cognitive functions.

6. Conclusions

Computerized cognitive assessments have come a long way in the past 35 years. The proliferation of technology has resulted in reliable and easy to administer batteries that have great potential for affecting how the health care system monitors and screens for cognitive changes in the aging population. Importantly, modern computerized and internet-based cognitive tasks have been designed to capitalize on the many advantages that computers can offer to create more efficient and accurate assessments than existing paper-and-pencil options. One of the key advantages is the way in which these tasks are scored and interpreted. Computerized tests can use statistical measures to interpret one individual's score within the context of thousands of normative data points and provide an objective interpretation of that individual's performance 'on-the-fly'. This shift moves away from the traditional intuition-based approach that more typically required a highly trained individual to interpret a constellation of test scores.

The objective nature of computerized test scores has implications for the adoption of these test batteries into health care because they do not need to be administered or interpreted by a highly trained individual. These batteries can be used by physicians, family members, or other front-line health care workers to monitor for subtle changes in cognition. Catching these changes and flagging them for a more thorough follow-up with the appropriate health-care professional helps to improve quality of life in patients with declining cognitive abilities as well as moves the responsibility of monitoring cognitive changes from a few highly trained individuals to a large number of front-line health-care providers. In short, self-administered online cognitive testing batteries have the potential to help close the dementia diagnosis gap without adding undue burden to the existing health care system.

Supplementary Materials: The following are available online at http://www.mdpi.com/2075-4418/9/3/114/s1.

Author Contributions: Conceptualization; writing–reviewing and editing, A.S., A.B., and A.M.O.; writing–original draft preparation, A.S.; funding acquisition, A.M.O.

Funding: This research was funded by the Canada Excellence Research Chairs Program (#215063), the Canadian Institutes of Health Research (#209907), and the Natural Sciences and Engineering Research Council of Canada (#390057).

Conflicts of Interest: The online cognitive tests (Cambridge Brain Sciences) discussed in this review are marketed by Cambridge Brain Sciences Inc, of which Dr. Owen is the unpaid Chief Scientific Officer. Under the terms of the existing licensing agreement, Dr. Owen and his collaborators are free to use the platform at no cost for their scientific studies and such research projects neither contribute to, nor are influenced by, the activities of the company. As such, there is no overlap between the current review and the activities of Cambridge Brain Sciences Inc, nor was there any cost to the authors, funding bodies or participants who were involved in the mentioned studies.

References

1. Harlow, J.M. Passage of an iron rod through the head. *Boston Med. Surg. J.* **1848**, *39*, 389–393. [CrossRef]
2. Cattell, J.M.; Farrand, L. Physical and mental measurements of the students of Columbia University. *Psychol. Rev.* **1896**, *3*, 618–648. [CrossRef]
3. Binet, A. *L'étude expérimentale de l'intelligence*; Schleicher frères & cie: Paris, France, 1903.
4. Wechsler, D. *Manual for the Wechsler Adult Intelligence Scale*; Psychological Corp.: Oxford, UK, 1955.
5. Wechsler, D. A standardized memory scale for clinical use. *J. Psychol.* **1945**, *19*, 87–95. [CrossRef]
6. Stroop, J.R. Studies of interference in serial verbal reactions. *J. Exp. Psychol.* **1935**, *18*, 643–662. [CrossRef]
7. Golden, C.J. *Stroop Color and Word Test: A Manual for Clinical and Experimental Uses*; Stoelting Co.: Wood Dale, IL, USA, 1978.
8. Folstein, M.F.; Folstein, S.E.; McHugh, P.R. "Mini-mental state". A practical method for grading the cognitive state of patients for the clinician. *J. Psychiatr. Res.* **1975**, *12*, 189–198. [CrossRef]
9. Bor, D.; Duncan, J.; Lee, A.C.H.; Parr, A.; Owen, A.M. Frontal lobe involvement in spatial span: Converging studies of normal and impaired function. *Neuropsychologia* **2006**, *44*, 229–237. [CrossRef]
10. Blackwell, A.D.; Sahakian, B.J.; Vesey, R.; Semple, J.M.; Robbins, T.W.; Hodges, J.R. Detecting Dementia: Novel Neuropsychological Markers of Preclinical Alzheimer's Disease. *Dement. Geriatr. Cogn. Disord.* **2003**, *17*, 42–48. [CrossRef]
11. Robbins, T.W.; James, M.; Owen, A.M.; Sahakian, B.J.; McInnes, L.; Rabbitt, P. Cambridge Neuropsychological Test Automated Battery (CANTAB): A Factor Analytic Study of a Large Sample of Normal Elderly Volunteers. *Dementia* **1994**, *5*, 266–281. [CrossRef]
12. Downes, J.J.; Roberts, A.C.; Sahakian, B.J.; Evenden, J.L.; Morris, R.G.; Robbins, T.W. Impaired extra-dimensional shift performance in medicated and unmedicated Parkinson's disease: Evidence for a specific attentional dysfunction. *Neuropsychologia* **1989**, *27*, 1329–1343. [CrossRef]
13. Morris, R.G.; Downes, J.J.; Sahakian, B.J.; Evenden, J.L.; Heald, A.; Robbins, T.W. Planning and spatial working memory in Parkinson's disease. *J. Neurol. Neurosurg. Psychiatry* **1988**, *51*, 757–766. [CrossRef]
14. Sahakian, B.J.; Owen, A.M. Computerized assessment in neuropsychiatry using CANTAB: discussion paper. *J. R. Soc. Med.* **1992**, *85*, 399–402.
15. Sahakian, B.J.; Morris, R.G.; Evenden, J.L.; Heald, A.; Levy, R.; Philpot, M.; Robbins, T.W. A comparative study of visuospatial memory and learning in Alzheimer-type dementia and Parkinson's Disease. *Brain* **1988**, *111*, 695–718. [CrossRef]
16. Sahakian, B.J.; Downes, J.J.; Eagger, S.; Everden, J.L.; Levy, R.; Philpot, M.P.; Roberts, A.C.; Robbins, T.W. Sparing of attentional relative to mnemonic function in a subgroup of patients with dementia of the Alzheimer type. *Neuropsychologia* **1990**, *28*, 1197–1213. [CrossRef]
17. Swainson, R.; Hodges, J.R.; Galton, C.J.; Semple, J.; Michael, A.; Dunn, B.D.; Iddon, J.L.; Robbins, T.W.; Sahakian, B.J. Early detection and differential diagnosis of Alzheimer's disease and depression with neuropsychological tasks. *Dement. Geriatr. Cogn. Disord.* **2001**, *12*, 265–280. [CrossRef]
18. Lee, A.C.H.; Rahman, S.; Hodges, J.R.; Sahakian, B.J.; Graham, K.S. Associative and recognition memory for novel objects in dementia: implications for diagnosis. *Eur. J. Neurosci.* **2003**, *18*, 1660–1670. [CrossRef]
19. Hampshire, A.; Highfield, R.R.; Parkin, B.L.; Owen, A.M. Fractionating Human Intelligence. *Neuron* **2012**, *76*, 1225–1237. [CrossRef]
20. Kane, R.; Roebuckspencer, T.; Short, P.; Kabat, M.; Wilken, J. Identifying and monitoring cognitive deficits in clinical populations using Automated Neuropsychological Assessment Metrics (ANAM) tests. *Arch. Clin. Neuropsychol.* **2007**, *22*, 115–126. [CrossRef]
21. Veroff, A.E.; Cutler, N.R.; Sramek, J.J.; Prior, P.L.; Mickelson, W.; Hartman, J.K. A new assessment tool for neuropsychopharmacologic research: the Computerized Neuropsychological Test Battery. *Top. Geriatr.* **1991**, *4*, 211–217. [CrossRef]
22. Inoue, M.; Jimbo, D.; Taniguchi, M.; Urakami, K. Touch Panel-type Dementia Assessment Scale: A new computer-based rating scale for Alzheimer's disease: A new computer-based rating scale for AD. *Psychogeriatrics* **2011**, *11*, 28–33. [CrossRef]

23. Wild, K.; Howieson, D.; Webbe, F.; Seelye, A.; Kaye, J. The status of computerized cognitive testing in aging: A systematic review. *Alzheimers Dement.* **2008**, *4*, 428–437. [CrossRef]

24. Zygouris, S.; Tsolaki, M. Computerized Cognitive Testing for Older Adults: A Review. *Am. J. Alzheimer's Dis. Other Dement.* **2015**, *30*, 13–28. [CrossRef]

25. Barnett, J.H.; Blackwell, A.D.; Sahakian, B.J.; Robbins, T.W. The Paired Associates Learning (PAL) Test: 30 Years of CANTAB Translational Neuroscience from Laboratory to Bedside in Dementia Research. *Curr. Top. Behav. Neurosci.* **2016**, *28*, 449–474.

26. Owen, A.M.; Hampshire, A.; Grahn, J.A.; Stenton, R.; Dajani, S.; Burns, A.S.; Howard, R.J.; Ballard, C.G. Putting brain training to the test. *Nature* **2010**, *465*, 775–778. [CrossRef]

27. Metzler-Baddeley, C.; Caeyenberghs, K.; Foley, S.; Jones, D.K. Task complexity and location specific changes of cortical thickness in executive and salience networks after working memory training. *NeuroImage* **2016**, *130*, 48–62. [CrossRef]

28. Pausova, Z.; Paus, T.; Abrahamowicz, M.; Bernard, M.; Gaudet, D.; Leonard, G.; Peron, M.; Pike, G.B.; Richer, L.; Séguin, J.R.; et al. Cohort Profile: The Saguenay Youth Study (SYS). *Int. J. Epidemiol.* **2017**, *46*, e19. [CrossRef]

29. Esopenko, C.; Chow, T.W.P.; Tartaglia, M.C.; Bacopulos, A.; Kumar, P.; Binns, M.A.; Kennedy, J.L.; Müller, D.J.; Levine, B. Cognitive and psychosocial function in retired professional hockey players. *J. Neurol. Neurosurg. Psychiatry* **2017**, *88*, 512–519. [CrossRef]

30. Nichols, E.S.; Wild, C.J.; Owen, A.M.; Soddu, A. Cognition across the lifespan: Aging and gender differences. *Cognition.* in submission.

31. Wild, C.J.; Nichols, E.S.; Battista, M.E.; Stojanoski, B.; Owen, A.M. Dissociable effects of self-reported daily sleep duration on high-level cognitive abilities. *Sleep* **2018**, *41*, 1–11. [CrossRef]

32. Schaie, K.; Maitland, S.B.; Willis, S.L.; Intrieri, R. Longitudinal invariance of adult psychometric ability factor structures across 7 years. *Psychol. Aging* **1998**, *13*, 8–20. [CrossRef]

33. Widaman, K.F.; Ferrer, E.; Conger, R.D. Factorial Invariance within Longitudinal Structural Equation Models: Measuring the Same Construct across Time. *Child. Dev. Perspect.* **2010**, *4*, 10–18. [CrossRef]

34. Honarmand, K.; Malik, S.; Wild, C.; Gonzalez-Lara, L.E.; McIntyre, C.W.; Owen, A.M.; Slessarev, M. Feasibility of a web-based neurocognitive battery for assessing cognitive function in critical illness survivors. *PLoS ONE* **2019**, *14*, e0215203. [CrossRef]

35. Stojanoski, B.; Lyons, K.M.; Pearce, A.A.A.; Owen, A.M. Targeted training: Converging evidence against the transferable benefits of online brain training on cognitive function. *Neuropsychologia* **2018**, *117*, 541–550. [CrossRef]

36. Nasreddine, Z.S.; Phillips, N.A.; Bédirian, V.; Charbonneau, S.; Whitehead, V.; Collin, I.; Cummings, J.L.; Chertkow, H. The Montreal Cognitive Assessment, MoCA: A brief screening tool for mild cognitive impairment. *J. Am. Geriatr. Soc.* **2005**, *53*, 695–699. [CrossRef]

37. Gluhm, S.; Goldstein, J.; Loc, K.; Colt, A.; Liew, C.V.; Corey-Bloom, J. Cognitive Performance on the Mini-Mental State Examination and the Montreal Cognitive Assessment Across the Healthy Adult Lifespan. *Cogn. Behav. Neurol.* **2013**, *26*, 1–5. [CrossRef]

38. Damian, A.M.; Jacobson, S.A.; Hentz, J.G.; Belden, C.M.; Shill, H.A.; Sabbagh, M.N.; Caviness, J.N.; Adler, C.H. The montreal cognitive assessment and the mini-mental state examination as screening instruments for cognitive impairment: Item analyses and threshold scores. *Dement. Geriatr. Cogn. Disord.* **2011**, *31*, 126–131. [CrossRef]

39. Malek-Ahmadi, M.; Powell, J.J.; Belden, C.M.; O'Connor, K.; Evans, L.; Coon, D.W.; Nieri, W. Age- and education-adjusted normative data for the Montreal Cognitive Assessment (MoCA) in older adults age 70–99. *Aging Neuropsychol. Cogn.* **2015**, *22*, 755–761. [CrossRef]

40. Brenkel, M.; Shulman, K.; Hazan, E.; Herrmann, N.; Owen, A.M. Assessing Capacity in the Elderly: Comparing the MoCA with a Novel Computerized Battery of Executive Function. *Dement. Geriatr. Cogn. Disord. Extra.* **2017**, *7*, 249–256. [CrossRef]

41. Levine, B.; Bacopulous, A.; Anderson, N.; Black, S.; Davidson, P.; Fitneva, S.; McAndrews, M.; Spaniol, J.; Jeyakumar, N.; Abdi, H.; et al. Validation of a Novel Computerized Test Battery for Automated Testing. In *Stroke*; Lippincott Williams & Wilkins: Philadelphia, PA, USA, 2013; Volume 44, p. 196.

42. Robbins, T.W.; James, M.; Owen, A.M.; Sahakian, B.J.; McInnes, L.; Rabbitt, P.; James, M.; Owen, A.M.; Sahakian, B.J.; McInnes, L.; et al. A Neural Systems Approach to the Cognitive Psychology of Ageing Using the CANTAB Battery. In *Methodology of Frontal and Executive Function*; Routledge: London, UK, 2004; pp. 216–239.

43. Yaffe, K.; Falvey, C.M.; Hoang, T. Connections between sleep and cognition in older adults. *Lancet Neurol.* **2014**, *13*, 1017–1028. [CrossRef]

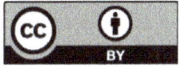

diagnostics

MDPI

Review

The Who, When, Why, and How of PET Amyloid Imaging in Management of Alzheimer's Disease—Review of Literature and Interesting Images

Subapriya Suppiah [1,2], Mellanie-Anne Didier [3,4] and Sobhan Vinjamuri [3,*]

1   Centre for Diagnostic Nuclear Imaging, University Putra Malaysia, Serdang 43400, Selangor, Malaysia;
    subapriya@upm.edu.my
2   Department of Imaging, Faculty of Medicine and Health Sciences, University Putra Malaysia, Serdang 43400,
    Selangor, Malaysia
3   The Royal Liverpool and Broadgreen University Hospitals NHS Trusts, Prescot St, Liverpool L7 8XP, UK;
    mellanie-anne.didier@rlbuht.nhs.uk
4   Section of Nuclear Medicine, Department of Surgery, Radiology, Anaesthesia & Intensive Care,
    The University Hospital of The West Indies, The University of The West Indies, Mona Campus,
    Kingston 7, Jamaica
*   Correspondence: Sobhan.Vinjamuri@rlbuht.nhs.uk

Received: 23 May 2019; Accepted: 21 June 2019; Published: 25 June 2019

Abstract: Amyloid imaging using positron emission tomography (PET) has an emerging role in the management of Alzheimer's disease (AD). The basis of this imaging is grounded on the fact that the hallmark of AD is the histological detection of beta amyloid plaques (Aβ) at post mortem autopsy. Currently, there are three FDA approved amyloid radiotracers used in clinical practice. This review aims to take the readers through the array of various indications for performing amyloid PET imaging in the management of AD, particularly using 18F-labelled radiopharmaceuticals. We elaborate on PET amyloid scan interpretation techniques, their limitations and potential improved specificity provided by interpretation done in tandem with genetic data such as apolipiprotein E (APO) 4 carrier status in sporadic cases and molecular information (e.g., cerebral spinal fluid (CSF) amyloid levels). We also describe the quantification methods such as the standard uptake value ratio (SUVr) method that utilizes various cutoff points for improved accuracy of diagnosing AD, such as a threshold of 1.122 (area under the curve 0.894), which has a sensitivity of 92.3% and specificity of 90.5%, whereas the cutoff points may be higher in APOE ε4 carriers (1.489) compared to non-carriers (1.313). Additionally, recommendations for future developments in this field are also provided.

Keywords: Alzheimer's disease; diagnostic imaging; molecular imaging; precision medicine; quantification; nuclear medicine; ^{18}F-FDG; PET; neurocognitive disorder

1. Introduction and Role of [^{18}F]FDG PET

Diagnostic imaging has always played an important role in the management of Alzheimer's disease (AD). Conventionally, neurologists and psychiatrists depended on magnetic resonance imaging (MRI) to help diagnose probable AD, particularly in atypical cases, by identifying typical anatomical changes that are characteristic of AD [1]. This type of structural imaging, however, has its limitations due to naturally occurring variations in brain volume caused by the aging process and co-existing conditions that can cause medial temporal lobe atrophy, such as depression [2]. Hence, functional imaging such as positron emission tomography (PET) offers an irresistible enticement for increased accuracy of diagnosis. PET is very important in providing a one-stop solution and its function is not limited only to the oncology field [3].

There are two main categories of radiopharmaceuticals that are utilized for PET/CT imaging in patients suspected with AD. Initially, 2-Deoxy-2-[^{18}F]fluorodeoxyglucose ([^{18}F]FDG), a glucose analog, was utilized for PET brain imaging for the management of AD. Healthy brain cells avidly take up the substance, as they highly metabolize glucose, but the substance is relatively reduced in uptake in the temporo-parietal cortical regions that are affected by AD. Although the role of [^{18}F]FDG has been established for making the diagnosis of AD, the accuracy of the scan interpretations can decline markedly when it involves older patients. In a younger cohort with a mean age of 64 years of age, the sensitivity of [^{18}F]FDG PET was reported to be 100%, with a specificity of 75% (accuracy 84%), whereas a study with older patients has reported 20% lower accuracy in late-onset AD [4]. Consequently, this limitation was the catalyst for the development of more specific biomarkers for the detection of AD, namely amyloid precursors. The detection of amyloid precursors is said to be able to predict the conversion of at risk subjects to full blown AD 10 years prior to the onset of AD symptoms [5].

Amyloid precursors for PET imaging such as the short radioactive half-life (20 minutes) Pittsburgh compound B ([^{11}C]PiB), by crossing the blood brain barrier (BBB) and selectively binding to beta amyloid plaques (Aβ), are able to provide a virtual ante mortem histopathological portrait of the brain. Similar but newer radiopharmaceuticals include ^{18}F-labeled Aβ targeting tracers, such as [^{18}F]Florbetapir (Amyvid, Eli Lilly, USA) ([^{18}F]FBP), [^{18}F]Florbetaben (Neuraceq, Piramal, Mumbai) ([^{18}F]FBB), and [^{18}F]Flutemetamol (Vizamyl GE Healthcare, USA) ([^{18}F]FMT) [6–9]. These amyloid radiotracers are more suited for clinical settings and have high specificity for the detection of Aβ plaques [10]. These are relatively novel radiopharmaceuticals used in the management of AD as they also enable the quantification of Aβ plaque burden in the brain cortices, which is a hallmark of AD.

Previous research has focused on [^{18}F]FDG PET studies as it is a widely available radiotracer for various imaging indications and has well established cutoff points for standardized uptake values (SUVs) utilized for disease process quantification. More specifically, [^{18}F]FDG PET is used to differentiate AD from other clinical diagnoses by normalizing the uptake intensity to the mean metabolic rate for glucose utilization in the whole brain (CMR$_{glc}$) or the cerebellar glucose consumption, as these areas allow for accurate distinction of AD, by being maximally stable in subjects but minimally affected by external stimuli and are relatively unaffected by the disease of interest [11]. Nevertheless, many factors influence the value of the measured glucose uptake, namely patient related factors such as fasting blood glucose levels and altered bio-distribution of [^{18}F]FDG [12]. Additionally, an inverse relationship has been noted between cortical retention of amyloid compared with cerebral glucose metabolism determined with [^{18}F]FDG, which was detected to be most robust in the posterior temporoparietal lobes [13]. This pathognomonic finding on [^{18}F]FDG PET, however, may be absent in certain cases and regional fibrillary amyloid depositions have been noted to have little to nil significant association with regional cortical FDG hypometabolism, but rather the impaired FDG metabolism is more influenced by global amyloid burden [14].

AD, which is a major neurocognitive disorder (NCD), was first described by Alois Alzheimer in 1906, by discovering intracerebral neuritic plaques and neurofibrillary tangles (NFTs) in the post mortem study of a patient with chronic mental illness [15]. AD is currently the most common NCD, with more than 36 million cases worldwide and nearly catastrophic in its prevalence among older adults [16]. As a matter of fact, the prevalence of AD after the age of 85 years old is 85 per 1000 population. Approximately 1% of AD is autosomal dominant inheritance due to mutations on chromosomes 21 (APP), 14 (presenilin 1), and 1 (presenilin 2), which leads to early onset familial Alzheimer's disease (oeFAD). Nevertheless, most cases are idiopathic and often the diagnosis is elusive until a later stage in the disease progression. There are several subtypes of neurocognitive disorders (NCDs) which include Alzheimer's disease (AD), dementia with Lewy bodies (DLB), vascular dementia (VaD), and fronto-temporal dementia (FTD). Some sufferers have mixed type of NCDs; however, AD is the commonest subtype with over 60% of subjects suffering from this disorder.

Diagnosis of AD is made primarily on the basis of clinical criteria using the Diagnostic and Statistical Manual, 4th and 5th editions (DSM-IV and DSM-5) [17]. This method is combined with neuropsychiatric testing to objectively assess for cognitive impairment, i.e., Mini Mental State Examination (MMSE) or the Montreal Cognitive Assessment (MoCA) scoring [18]. For instance, in the absence of secondary causes, using MMSE scoring helps to grade the severity of cognitive decline with subjects scoring < 15/30 as having severe AD, < 24/30 being more likely to have mild AD, as well as subjects with reported memory deficits, and normal or slightly low scores but preserved ADL (activities of daily living), of having mild cognitive impairment (MCI) [17]. Moreover, subject education level has to be factored in when interpreting the assessment score. A set of standards created in 1984 by the National Institute of Neurological and Communicative Disorders and Stroke (NINCDS) and the Alzheimer's disease and Related Disorders Association (ADRDA) known as the NINCDS-ADRDA criteria had a sensitivity of 81% and specificity of 70% of diagnosing AD [19]. However, due to new developments in the field, Knopman et al., proposed recommendations in 2001 [20], which were later revised in 2011 [21].

The National Institute on Aging-Alzheimer's Association (NIA-AA) workgroups involved in preparation of diagnostic guidelines for AD, set a revised guideline that took into account distinguishing features of other dementing/neurocognitive deficit causing conditions that occur in a similarly aged population, which were not completely recognized in the past [21]. These criteria could help differentiate NCD subtypes such as DLB, VaD, and FTD from AD, as they have inherently different clinical characteristics, as well as unique pathophysiological features. The criteria propose the use of two classes of biomarkers to help diagnose AD, namely biomarkers for brain amyloid Aβ protein deposition detection and the biomarkers for downstream neuronal injury identification [21]. The former class includes two major biomarkers namely detection of reduced cerebrospinal fluid (CSF) Aβ$_{42}$ levels and positive PET amyloid imaging, whereas the latter includes three major biomarkers, namely elevated CSF tau, reduced [^{18}F]FDG uptake on PET in the temporoparietal lobes, and disproportionate atrophy at the medial, basal, and lateral temporal lobes on structural MRI scans [21]. Nevertheless, the criteria have their limitations with regards to absolute classification of subtypes due to the presence of certain inherent heterogeneity within the groups. For example, it is difficult to differentiate NCD subjects who have tauopathy disorders such as FTD, progressive supranuclear palsy (PSP), and cortico-basal degeneration [22].

In addition, the International Working Group (IWG) and the US NIA-AA have contributed criteria for the diagnosis of AD that better define clinical phenotypes and integrate the role of neuroimaging, genetic profiling, and CSF biomarkers [23]. Some of the recommendations are stated as a guideline and others are given as an option to be utilized at the discretion of the clinician. At present it is accepted that a good clinical assessment yields fairly good sensitivity and specificity to diagnose the different subtypes of NCDs and is reasonably on par with other types of investigations to diagnose AD. The IWG has proposed revisions to the diagnostic algorithm for defining typical and atypical AD, identifying mixed type of AD and preclinical states of AD [23].

The objective of this review is to expound on the various arrays of indications for performing amyloid PET imaging in the management of AD, how to interpret the scans, and the limitations of the test. PET quantification methods used to assess Aβ plaque load in the brain will also be clarified.

2. The Role of PET Amyloid Imaging in the Management of AD

There are various radiotracers that have been experimented with to enable in vivo detection of amyloid depositions in the brain. Among the main indications for performing an amyloid scan is to confirm the diagnosis in indeterminate or atypical cases, to aid in early detection of AD among subjects with mild cognitive impairment (MCI) and to enable quantification of progressive changes in brain amyloid load in response to anti-amyloid therapy. Currently, there are several compounds detected to have a high affinity to bind with fibrillary Aβ plaques that have received FDA approval. There is also a newer benzofuran derivative for the imaging of Aβ in vivo, i.e., [18F]FPYBF-2 (5-(5-(2-(2-(2-18F-fluoroethoxy)ethoxy)ethoxy)benzofuran-2-yl)-N-methylpyridin-2-amine), which is chemically stable, does not photodegrade, and has been tested for feasibility in distinguishing AD patients [24].

2.1. [¹¹C]Pittsburgh Compound-B

In January 2004, Klunk et al. published the first human amyloid PET study using ¹¹C-labeled Pittsburgh Compound-B ([¹¹C]PiB), also known as 2-(4-N-[¹¹C]methylaminophenyl)-6-hydroxybenzothiazole. This compound, which is radiolabeled to ¹¹C, has approximately 20-minutes half-life. Therefore, its use is restricted to centres that have an on-site cyclotron facility. Compared with healthy controls, AD patients typically showed marked retention of [¹¹C]PiB in areas of cerebral cortex that have been identified to contain substantial amounts of deposition of fibrillar Aβ plaques in AD patients [25]. Interestingly, an inverse relationship was noted between [¹¹C]PiB cortical retention with cerebral glucose metabolism determined with [¹⁸F]FDG, which was most prominent in the parietal lobes [25].

Using distribution volume ratio (DVR) method, Rowe et al. demonstrated that there was higher [¹¹C]PiB binding in neocortical areas in AD and DLB patients when compared with healthy control subjects, and no cortical binding in FTD [26]. Although almost all AD patients have significantly positive [¹¹C]PiB scans, especially in later stages of the disease, even healthy adults can have falsely positive scan results, e.g., up to 12% of adults in their 60s, 30% of adults in their 70s, and a minimum of 50% of adults in their 80s [26]. The annual incidence of healthy subjects to develop [¹¹C]PiB positivity, as reported in a publication from the Mayo Clinic, evaluating elderly population, was estimated to be 13% per year [27].

2.2. [¹⁸F]Florbetapir Scan

[¹⁸F]Florbetapir ([¹⁸F]FBP), which is also known as ¹⁸F-AV-45 or 4-{(E)-2-[6-(2-{2-[2-(18F)Fluoroethoxy]ethoxy}ethoxy)-3-pyridinyl]vinyl}-N-methylaniline, is an ¹⁸F-labelled amyloid PET ligand that has high accuracy in detecting brain amyloid deposition [28]. It is taken up rapidly through the BBB, and rapidly washed out from grey matter tissue that does not contain amyloid. It has a high affinity to aggregated Aβ, good separation between the radiotracer amyloid retention and background signal, and a long, stable pseudo-equilibrium allowing flexibility in the timing of image acquisition [29]. [¹⁸F]FBP received the U.S. FDA approval in 2012, to be the initial nuclear medicine imaging radiotracer allowed to be utilized for subjects who are being investigated for AD or other causes of cognitive decline [30]. It has an advantage over [¹¹C]PiB because it has a longer half-life, which is approximately 110 min that makes it possible to transport it from site of production to regional PET scanner facilities.

It also demonstrates excellent specificity to Aβ detection and has favorable pharmacokinetics, whereby it is quickly cleared from the blood circulation with approximately 10% of the radiotracer remaining at 20 min post injection. The radiotracer readily enters the brain and 20 min post injection, a clear separation can be seen between individuals with and without significant cerebral amyloid deposition (Figure 1).

[¹⁸F]FBP is maximally taken up in the brains of subjects with presumed presence of aggregated fibrillar Aβ after 30 min post injection. Furthermore, its biodistribution is stable for up to 60 min of being introduced intravenously. This allows a wide time window to facilitate the recommended imaging protocol of 10 min. Radiation dosimetry assessments in humans have indicated that the highest organ exposures to the introduced amyloid radioligand occur in the liver, gallbladder, urinary bladder, and the gut [28].

It is noteworthy that a significant amount of amyloid burden has been detected in [¹⁸F]FBP scans among even cognitively normal elderly patients who have uncontrolled hypertension and underlying risk factors such as the presence of one or more APOE ε4 alleles [31]. Nevertheless, [¹⁸F]FBP is widely used as a research biomarker in the Alzheimer's Disease Neuroimaging Initiative (ADNI) project and in several phase III clinical trials of experimental AD drugs.

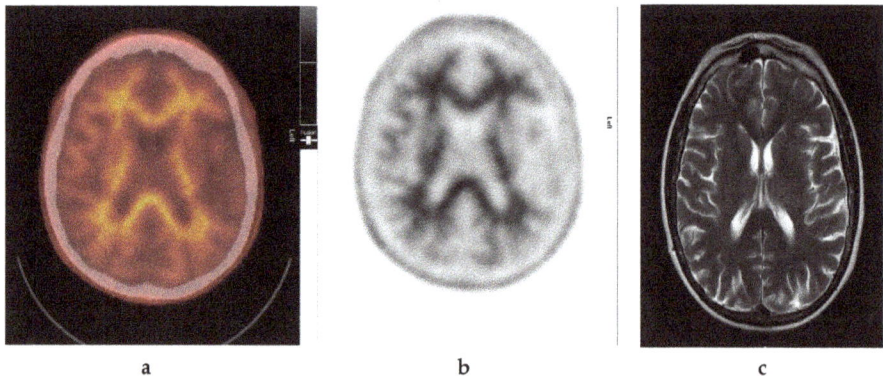

Figure 1. Normal study. Sixty-seven year old female patient with deteriorating cognition and multiple vascular risk factors for assessment for vascular dementia. (**a**) and (**b**) [18F]FBP shows good contrast between grey and white matter in all sections of the brain with no obvious evidence of beta amyloid plaque disease. This suggests that the diagnosis/development of Alzheimer's disease is less likely. (**c**) MRI brain scan (multiplanar and multi sequence acquisitions) shows no significant T2 signal abnormality or restricted diffusion to suggest space occupying lesion, infarction, or ischemic change. (figures are courtesy RLBUHT Hospital database).

2.3. [^{18}F]Florbetaben

[^{18}F]Florbetaben ([^{18}F]FBB) is another radiotracer used in amyloid PET imaging. In a study carried out in 2012 by Villemagne et al. [^{11}C]PiB and [^{18}F]FBB images were co-registered so that the selection of regions of interest (ROIs) were similar in both scans [32]. This was followed by utilizing the cerebellar cortex as a region of reference to calculate the standard uptake value ratios (SUVr). This gave good concordance of elevated SUVr using [^{18}F]FBB in subjects with AD compared to healthy controls [32].

2.4. [^{18}F]Flutemetamol

[^{18}F]Flutemetamol ([^{18}F]FMT) is a PET radiotracer with an extended half-life, which enables it to be distributed in vivo for a longer duration compared to [^{18}F]FBP. The data indicate that, as an amyloid imaging agent, the performance of [^{18}F]FMT is similar to that of [^{11}C]PiB in AD and AD-associated MCI [32]. Furthermore, a comparison made among amyloid radiotracers [^{11}C]PiB, [^{18}F]FBP, and [^{18}F]FMT revealed good contrast between composite amyloid retention ratio that was normalized by whole cerebellum, along with consistent detection of Aβ positivity in the scans [33].

3. The Role of PET Using Tau Imaging Radioligands

PET imaging that detects tau proteins is able to differentiate AD from other types of NCDs, namely DLB. The PET ligand [^{18}F]AV-1451 (formerly known as T807) binds to a broad spectrum of tau-positive inclusions, but not to tau-negative aggregates in autopsy samples from NCDs other than AD. In 2015, Rabinovici et al. reported preliminary in vivo results applying [^{18}F]AV-1451 PET imaging to patients with NCDs other than AD, which were associated with positive or negative tau pathology with promising results [34]. Additionally, [^{18}F]Florbenazine (^{18}F-AV-133), which is a biomarker for vesicular monoamine type 2 transporters (VMAT2), has been noted to be significantly decreased in the Parkinson's disease/DLB group compared to AD patients, and can help to differentiate the two conditions in atypical cases. Neurocognitive impairment in DLB patients is significantly associated with VMAT2 density. Furthermore, significant differences have been detected in consecutive [^{18}F]AV-133 and [18F]FBP scans that are consistent with expected NCD pathology, i.e., greater amyloid depositions in AD and DLB as compared with Parkinson's disease and controls [35].

4. Enabling Early and Accurate Diagnosis of AD

In as much as AD progression is attributed to three cardinal neuropathological features, i.e., deposition of senile plaques in the extracellular matrix, neurofibrillary tangles (NFTs) accumulated in the intracellular compartment and synaptic degeneration, it is believed that it is actually the fibrillary Aβ particles that are crucial for the ultimate dysfunction of neurons and development of AD [36]. Although Aβ pathology is consistently detected in post mortem studies of AD patients, it has been reported to be present in 25–45% of normal elderly individuals [37]. This finding depends on the age of the cohort and the pathological criteria employed. It has been suggested that the presence of this pathology reflects the earliest stage in the development of AD [38]. Proving this hypothesis is a real challenge, caused by limitations inherent in post mortem analysis. Fortunately, recent developments of functional amyloid imaging that binds to fibrillar Aβ plaques, provides a unique opportunity to quantify this pathology in the ante mortem state.

[^{18}F]FBP, [^{18}F]FBB, and [^{18}F]FMT all have good affinity to bind with Aβ plaques, and are potentially excellent non-invasive tools for in vivo imaging of NCDs. In familial hereditary AD, significant brain amyloid burden appears years before symptoms of NCD [39], plus accumulation of amyloid deposits may start earlier than in sporadic AD. Amyloid imaging, particularly using the cerebellar grey matter or cerebral grey matter, has the potential clinical utility for aiding in differential diagnosis in early-onset AD and to support the clinical diagnosis of subjects with probable AD with improved diagnostic accuracy [1,40–44] (Table 1).

Alzheimer's Association and the Society of Nuclear Medicine and Molecular Imaging convened the Amyloid Imaging Taskforce (AIT) to gather empirical evidence that can help support the clinical utility of amyloid imaging. The AIT agreed upon a set of specific appropriate use criteria (AUC), ultimately empowering authorized medical practitioners to identify the types of patients and clinical circumstances in which amyloid PET could be used. It is recommended that patients who have persistent unexplained MCI, patients with atypical presentations of AD, and patients at an atypically early age who develop progressive NCD symptoms are more likely to benefit from this test [45]. As it is a very sub-specialized imaging tool, it is recommended that AD experts decide on the patients that would best benefit from an amyloid scan. The expert for this purpose should be self-identified as a physician trained and board-certified in neurology, psychiatry, or geriatric medicine who actively devotes a substantial proportion (≥25%) of patient contact time to the evaluation and care of adults with acquired mild cognitive impairment (MCI) or AD, as confirmed by peer recognition [45].

Although almost all AD patients have significantly positive amyloid scans, especially in the later stages of life, even cognitively normal elderly adults can have falsely positive scan results, which acts as a caveat for the interpretation of positive amyloid scans. Notably, the annual incidence of healthy subjects becoming amyloid scan positive, as reported in a recent study from the Mayo Clinic, evaluating elderly subjects, was estimated to be 13% per year [27].

5. Prognostication of Disease and Detecting Potential MCI Converters

In patients who are diagnosed with MCI, it may be beneficial to perform amyloid PET imaging to assess the plaque burden. This imaging has been known to detect high plaque burden, which can indicate a higher chance of the individual to convert to AD. Furthermore, many recent studies postulate that perhaps imaging is not a stand-alone test and the addition of CSF biomarkers, genetic information, and glucose metabolism to aid in the diagnosis may help improve the accuracy of interpretation of results [24,46–49] (Table 2). The role of amyloid PET imaging in MCI subjects has been extensively researched with variable results. Nevertheless, it is important to note that amyloid imaging is contraindicated in asymptomatic individuals because there are potentially more harmful than beneficial effects on the subject due to inaccurate assumptions made about the risks of developing AD and future outcomes on the basis of scan results per se.

Table 1. Clinical utility of amyloid positron emission tomography (PET) scans in diagnosing Alzheimer's disease (AD).

Author (Year)	Amyloid Tracer	Subjects	Age	Dose of Tracer (MBq)	Uptake Time (min)	Clinical Ref.	Reference Standard	Findings
Chiang (2017) [40]	[11C]PiB	Cognitively healthy older adults	63 ± 5	555	60	DSM-5	MRS at hippocampus PiB: Cerebellar GM	Corrected for APOE ε3/ε4 positivity: ↓ glutathione levels associated with ↑ amyloid load at the hippocampus
Chiaravalloti (2018) [41]	[18F]FBB, [18F]FDG	AD: 38, Control FDG: 58	AD: 69 ± 8	[18F]FBB: 295–320, FDG: 185–210	[18F]FBB: 90	MMSE: 21.7 ± 5.9	ROI placed at selected cortical GM	FDG hypo-metabolism correlated with Amyloid positivity at temporal, parietal and limbic regions. Mean normalised SUV: 1.28 +/− 0.1
Ciarmiello (2019) [42]	[18F]FBB	66 (MCI)	75.97 ± 6.59	306 ± 29	86 ± 8	MMSE 25.4 ± 3.07	cerebellar GM	SUVr 1.3 = positive scan, 54% of positive scans correlated with AD neuropathology among MCI
Miki (2017) [43]	[18F]FMT	Total: 70 AD: 25 MCI: 20 Controls: 25	75 ± 6	Single dose: 185 Cumulative dose: 240	90	NINCDS-ARDRA DSM-IV	Cerebellar GM	Visual reads: PPV: 88–92% NPV: 96–100%
Pothier (2019) [44]	[18F]FBP	Cognitively normal older adults: 65 (MCI: 31, Controls: 34)	76.11 years old ± 4.73	4 MBq/kg body weight	50	MMSE, CDR	cerebellar GM	visual reads: Aβ+ > 1.21, SUVr cutoffs: Aβ+ > 1.17, Aβ− < 1.10, equivocal amyloid load as in between range. no significant difference in cognitive decline in Aβ+ and Aβ− groups
Suppiah (2018) [1]	[18F]FBP	47 (Probable AD: 17, Possible AD: 30)	Probable AD: 63.5 ± 9.2, Possible AD: 62.7 ± 10.7	370	30	DSM-5, MMSE	visual reads of global cortical uptake compared with cerebellar GM	sensitivity: 62.5%, specificity: 77.4%, PPV: 58.8% NPV:80.0%, severity of amyloid load was not correlated with diagnosis of probable AD

[18F]FBB: Florbetaben, APOE: apolipoprotein genotype, AD: Alzheimer's disease, MCI: mild cognitive impairment (particularly amnestic type), CDR: Clinical Dementia Rating scale, Aβ+: amyloid beta positive PET scans, Aβ−: amyloid beta negative PET scans, NINCDS-ADRDA: National Institute of Neurological and Communicative Disorders and Stroke and the Alzheimer's disease and Related Disorders Association, WM: white matter, GM: grey matter, Aβ42/40: CSF amyloid beta 42/40 ratio, ROI: region of interest, SUVr: standardized uptake value ratio, ref.: reference, DSM: Diagnostic and Statistical Manual, PPV: positive predictive value, NPV: negative predictive value, MRS: MRI spectroscopy.

Table 2. Amyloid PET findings correlated with other biomarkers of AD and mild cognitive impairment (MCI).

Author (Year)	Amyloid Tracer	Other Biomarkers	Subjects	Age (Years)	Dose of Tracer (MBq)	Uptake Time (min)	Clinical Reference	Reference Standard	Findings
Alongi (2019) [46]	[18F]FBB	CSF amyloid levels	44 (neuro-cognitive deficit)	AD: 72.3, Controls: 68	269 ± 10%	90	ENS-EFNS criteria, MMSE	cerebellar WM	SUVr highest at precuneus, Amyloid PET: sens: 90.9%, spec: 78.9%, CSF amyloid <750 pg/mL: sens: 81.5% spec: 75.9%
Bouter (2019) [47]	[18F]FBB	CSF amyloid levels	33 (neuro-cognitive deficit)	68.4 ± 10.3	300	90	MMSE 25.2 ± 3.0	global cortex	↓Aβ42/40 & SUVr correlated with MMSE, mean SUVr: APOE ε4 carrier: 1.489, non-carriers: 1.313
Frings (2018) [48]	[11C]PiB	[18F]FDG	39 (MCI)	Converter: 69.8 ± 7.1 Non converter: 70.0 ± 6.4	[11C]PiB: 393 ± 56 [18F] FDG: 224 ± 36	[18F]FDG: 50-70	NINCDS-ADRDA	cerebellar GM	[11C]PiB PET predicted conversion from MCI to AD, HR for positive [11C]PiB scan: 10.2 (95% CI 1.3-78.1)
Higashi (2018) [24]	[18F]FPYBF-2	[11C]PiB	Controls: 61. Cases with suspected AD: 55 (AD: 27, MCI: 16, CN: 3, other NCDs: 9)	Controls: 53.7 ± 13.1, Cases: 74.4 ± 9.4	200 ± 22	50-70	DSM-IV and DSM-5 NINCDS-ADRDA	cerebellar GM	good correlation of PiB with [18F]FPYBF-2, Mean Cortical Index: early AD: 1.288 ± 0.134 moderate AD: 1.342 ± 0.191, PiB SUVr: 1.435 ± 0.474
Kim (2018) [49]	[18F]FBB, [18F]FMT	APOE	523 (MCI) Aβ+: 238 Aβ-: 285	Validation Set Aβ+: 71.4 ± 7.2 Aβ-: 69.7 ± 8.2	[18F]FBB: 311.5 [18F]FMT: 197.7	90	DSM-IV and DSM-5, Seoul Neuro-psycho-logical Screening Battery	Visuals reads based on uptake at selected ROI	Positivity for APOE ε4 (OR 4.14) among MCI is associated with PET Aβ+.

[18F]FBB: Florbetaben, [18F]FMT: [18F]-Flutemetamol, APOE: apolipoprotein genotype, AD: Alzheimer's disease, MCI: mild cognitive impairment (particularly amnestic type), CN: cognitively normal by neurophychiatric tests, Aβ+: amyloid beta positive PET scans, Aβ−: amyloid beta negative PET scans, ENS-EFNS: European Federation of the Neurological Societies dementia Guidelines, NINCDS-ADRDA: National Institute of Neurological and Communicative Disorders and Stroke and the Alzheimer's disease and Related Disorders Association, WM: white matter, GM: grey matter, Aβ42/40: CSF amyloid beta 42/40 ratio, ROI: region of interest, SUVr: standardized uptake value ratio, HR: hazard ratio, [18F]FDG: [18F]-Fluorodeoxyglucose, DSM: Diagnostic and Statistical Manual, [18F]FPYBF-2: 5-(5-(2-(2-(2-[18F]-fluoroethoxy)ethoxy)benzofuran-2-yl)-N-methylpyridin-2-amine.

6. Aiding in Treatment Planning and Monitoring

Amyloid PET neuroimaging can act as a surrogate biomarker for the assessment of neuronal function and integrity. It can be utilized to quantify the beta amyloid peptide plaque burden in the cortices of the brain [1]. The development of this radiotracer has enabled works related to the formulation of disease-modifying drugs that can dissolve the intracerebral amyloid plaques. Hence, this type of targeted neuroimaging can act as a quantitative biomarker for the assessment of treatment response.

7. Pharmacokinetics of Amyloid Tracers and Scanning Protocol

Amyloid radioligands demonstrate high affinity and specificity to Aβ and favorable pharmacokinetics. The tracer, particularly [^{18}F]FBP (approximately 370 Mbq or 10 mci), is injected intravenously [1], followed by approximately 30–50 min uptake time, some radioligands such as [18F]FMT may require 90 min and others such as [18F]FBB may require up to 130 min to achieve equilibrium [40]. The image acquisition time is commonly 10 min. The compounds are rapidly cleared from circulation with only 10% remaining 20 min after injection. The substances readily enter the brain and 20 min post injection, a clear separation can be seen between individuals with and without amyloid (Figures 2–4).

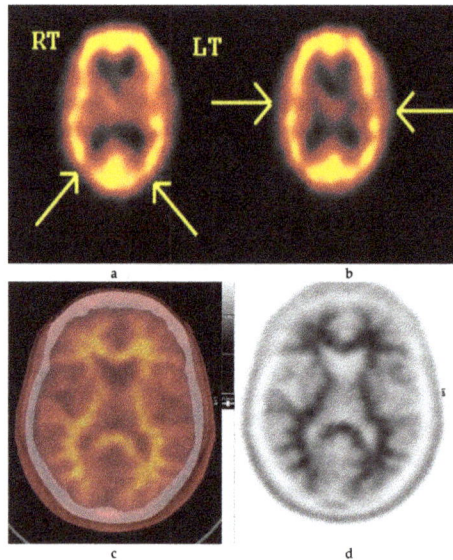

Figure 2. Normal study. Fifty-seven year old female patient memory problems/loss and confusion with a query of Alzheimer's disease. (**a**) and (**b**) Technetium-99m HMPAO-SPECT brain Scan [^{99m}Tc]HMPAO-SPECT brain scan. Brain scan showed mildly reduced perfusion to both temporal and both parietal lobes (yellow arrows) with relatively better perfusion anteriorly. Reduction of cerebral blood flow in these regions is commonly seen in patients with early Alzheimer's dementia rather than vascular dementia. However, in view of the subtle nature of the appearances on the [^{99m}Tc]HMPAO-SPECT brain scan, the [^{18}F]FBP brain scan was performed to identify beta amyloid plaque disease and to give a higher confidence for AD diagnosis or suggest vascular aetiology. (**c**) Color coded [^{18}F]FBP scan. (**d**) Grey scale [^{18}F]FBP scan shows good contrast between grey and white matter in sections of the brain and no obvious evidence of beta amyloid plaque disease. This means that the likelihood of developing AD is low and as such the overall findings are more suggestive of vascular aetiology rather than early AD. (Figures are courtesy RLBUHT Hospital database).

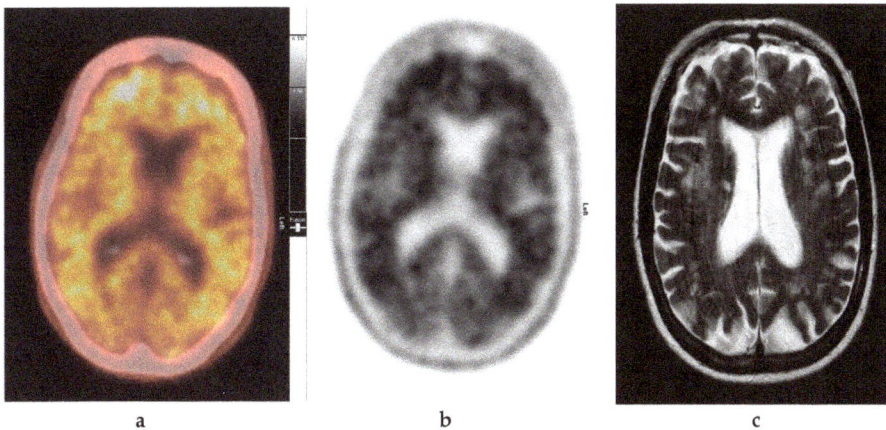

Figure 3. Abnormal study. Seventy-four year old male patient with a history of short term memory problems/gradual memory decline for some time and a query of dementing pathology. (**a**) and (**b**) [18F]FBP shows loss of contrast between grey and white matter in all sections of the brain. The scan is suggestive of beta-amyloid plaque deposition and in a patient with the above clinical presentation is suggestive of early AD. (**c**) MRI brain scan (multiplanar and multi sequence acquisitions) with some motion artefact shows generalised age appropriate cerebral atrophy, proportionate symmetrical temporal lobe atrophy, and corresponding dilatation of the cerebrospinal fluid (CSF) spaces. Moderate to marked periventricular T2 white matter hyperintensities likely to represent chronic small vessel ischemic changes. No diffusion restriction or space occupying lesions were identified. (Figures are courtesy RLBUHT Hospital database.).

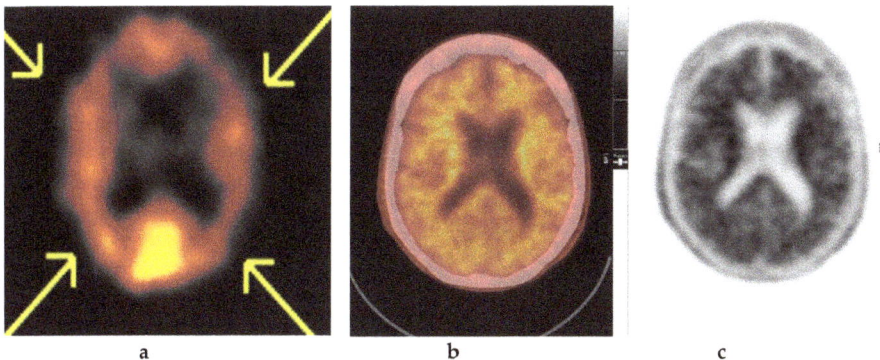

Figure 4. Abnormal study. Sixty-eight year old female patient with speech difficulties, deficits in memory, and visuospatial abilities. (**a**) [^{99m}Tc]HMPAO-SPECT brain scan shows asymmetrical heterogenous reduced perfusion to both parietal and temporal lobes (worse on the left side) as with involvement of the frontal lobes identified by the yellow arrows. Normal areas of temporal perfusion were noted in between the abnormal parietal and frontal areas. In a patient with cognitive impairment, the findings indicate patterns of cerebral blood flow commonly seen in patients with mixed dementia, i.e., Alzheimer's disease with vascular dementia. (**b**) Color coded [^{18}F]FBP scan. (**c**) Grey scale [^{18}F]FBP scans show loss of contrast between grey and white matter in all sections of the brain suggestive of beta-amyloid plaque deposition/disease. In conjunction with the [^{99m}Tc]HMPAO-SPECT brain scan, the overall findings are again suggestive of vascular as well as beta amyloid plaque disease (early AD), making the diagnosis mixed type AD. (Figures are courtesy RLBUHT Hospital database).

In brains presumed to have aggregated Aβ, maximum uptake of [18F]FBP occurs approximately 30 min after injection and remains essentially unchanged for the subsequent 60 min, thus providing a wide time window to facilitate the 10-minute imaging protocol. Whole-body radiation dosimetry studies in humans indicate the pathway for excretion of the radioligand, with the gallbladder, intestines, liver, and urinary bladder demonstrating the highest exposure [28].

8. In Vivo Assessment and Measurement of Cerebral Amyloid Burden

The clinical use of amyloid PET commonly relies on visual assessment and interpretation (VA) of scans, in which the signal intensity of "target-rich" brain regions such as the frontal cortex is contrasted to that of "target-poor" regions such as subcortical white matter (Figure 2). VA can be used for assessing the likelihood of significant fibrillar Aβ burden in the brain. A systematic qualitative VA of images is necessary, so that evidence of standardized interpretation protocols that lead to acceptable levels of inter-rater agreement can be achieved. The interpretation of amyloid scans needs to be conducted by an imaging expert, to determine the presence or absence of Aβ plaque deposition. The imaging expert is usually a nuclear medicine specialist or radiologist with specific training in the interpretation of amyloid PET [45]. The amyloid PET data must be technically adequate and must be acquired at a fully qualified and certified facility for it to be of diagnostic quality.

The criteria for interpreting the [18F]FBP scan as positive for AD by the VA method is identifying the presence of amyloid binding in the cortical regions relative to the cerebellum, which gives a poor grey-white matter contrast in the affected cerebral cortex. Among the brain areas affected by familial type of AD, which is related to the presence of amyloid precursor protein (APP) and Presenilin gene mutations, the striatal regions have been reported to have the highest amyloid depositions [50]. Sporadic type of AD that is related to APOE ε4 carrier status does not seem to have any regional predilection for amyloid burden; however, the amyloid deposition tends to have an earlier appearance in ApoE epsilon 4 carriers than non-carriers [50]. In a study performed by Newberg et al., [18F]FDG PET scans were interpreted as positive if they displayed the classic pattern of hypometabolism in the temporo-parietal regions [51]. Based on that criterion, scans were classified as either positive or negative for AD. In addition, relative scoring systems have been used to assess the degree of either FDG hypometabolism or increased amyloid binding characteristic of specified regions based on a priori knowledge. Cluster analysis by La Joie et al. revealed distinct subsets of regions [52]:

1. in the hippocampus, atrophy exceeded hypometabolism, whereas Aβ load was minimal,
2. in posterior association areas, Aβ deposition was predominant, together with high hypometabolism and lower but still significant atrophy, and
3. in frontal regions, Aβ deposition was maximal, whereas detection of structural and metabolic alterations was low.

Atrophy and hypometabolism significantly correlated in the hippocampus and temporo-parietal cortex, whereas Aβ load was not significantly related to either atrophy or hypometabolism. Thus, they postulated that these findings probably reflect the differential involvement of region-specific pathological or protective mechanisms, such as the presence of neurofibrillary tangles (NFTs), disconnection, as well as compensation processes.

9. Quantitative Interpretation of Cortical Aβ

The quantitative assessment of amyloid plaques requires consistent efforts for standardization of protocols. The steps involved include proper subject selection and management, calibrated dosage of radiotracer administration, image analysis and quality control, selection of brain reference region, and optimization of various image processing and segmentation methods [50]. Technical factors can be attributed to lead to variability in measurements, and can affect interpretation of the scans, e.g., scanner parameters, injected dose, movement correction methods, and uptake time.

Among the regions of the brain that have the lowest fibrillary amyloid plaques are the cerebellar white matter and almost none in the cerebellar grey matter. Thus, these regions are preferentially used to calculate SUVr values. Particularly, the cerebellar cortex was selected as a reference standard for the very first clinical study using [^{11}C]PiB PET due to its absence of Congo red and thioflavin-S stained plaques [51]. In addition, the clearance of amyloid radiotracers from cerebellar grey matter is considered more similar to its clearance from the cerebral grey matter target regions [52]. Similarly, Schmidt et al. described quantitative assessment of cortical amyloid signal (reflecting amyloid plaque deposition) relative to a reference region that is believed not to accumulate amyloid (normal reference area), producing the SUVr measurement [50]. Wong et al. employed parametric reference region method or a simplified SUVr calculated from 10 min of scanning, 50–60 min after [^{18}F]FBP administration [29].

A step by step approach at assessment of amyloid scans is to scrutinize the CT scan images for abnormalities in the structure. Subsequently, ROIs will be selected to evaluate cortical regions associated with significant amyloid burden in MCI and AD patients. By using the Montreal Neurological Institute (MNI) atlas on SPM software the scans are normalized to the standard brain template and mean cortical and cerebellar values are calculated to give the SUVr data. Routinely, six (6) cortical grey matter regions are targeted for the ROI analysis, i.e., anterior and posterior cingulate, medial orbital frontal, temporal, and parietal lobes, and the precuneus [53].

There have been many preset threshold SUVr values that have been proposed to improve the sensitivity and specificity of amyloid PET scans (Table 1, column 8 and Table 2, column 9). Among the initially recommended preset cutoff points of SUVr ≥ 1.17 was indicated to reflect amyloid levels in the pathological range based on separate in vivo PET studies and autopsy reports from nineteen (19) end-of-life patients [54]. Hence, they were able to portray that [^{18}F]FBP PET SUVr values can potentially be used to characterize fibrillary amyloid levels in clinical cases having probable AD, MCI, and among cognitively normal older adults, by using continuous and binary visual read measures of Aβ load. Frequently, concurrent MRI scans are used to normalize the PET data and improve on the anatomical localization of AD pathology.

Conversely, qualitative visual reads assessment using amyloid PET scans have been noted to have a sensitivity of approximately 84.6% (95% CI 0.55–0.98) and a specificity of approximately 38.1% (95% CI 0.18–0.62) for differentiating AD patients from healthy control subjects [55]. Nevertheless, improved scan parameters and the combination of other biomarkers have aided in improving the test accuracy (Table 1; Table 2). Although the quantitative assessment of the global cortex SUVr—despite being more time consuming—is advocated to be more accurate, with improved sensitivity of 92.3% and specificity of 90.5% using a threshold value of 1.122 (area under the curve, AUC 0.894) [55], much work is needed for the standardization of scanning and the reporting techniques, the protocol for global regional uptake assessment, and the selection of the region of reference.

In view of visual assessment and SUVr assessment having a discrepancy of approximately 10%, it is evident that we need to look elsewhere for further improvements in the diagnostic confidence of interpreting amyloid PET scans. Quantification is particularly useful in equivocal cases and for the purpose of providing numerical data that can reflect the change in amyloid load that is related to anti-amyloid therapy.

Finally, it is important to be aware that AD occurs as a spectrum of impairment in various levels of cognitive function, sometimes with additional confounding neuropsychiatric symptoms, which makes it difficult to have a standardized tool or threshold for confirming the diagnosis. As a matter of fact, it is well known that there are discordant areas of sites of atrophy noted on structural MRI, regional hypometabolism noted on ^{18}F-FDG PET with areas of amyloid deposition detected by amyloid PET imaging. This phenomenon is likely due to the longitudinal evolution of hypometabolism, which occurs in the cerebral regions that are remotely located but connected by functionality with areas of increased amyloid burden [56]. Hence, it is evident that various imaging data, clinical, molecular, and genetic information are required to be evaluated in tandem as they provide complementary information for improved management of AD.

10. Limitations

The prevalence of amyloid PET positivity among healthy older adults is among the main limitations of this diagnostic imaging. It is speculated that age-specific positivity rates for amyloid PET are less than 5% in those 50–60 years old, 10–12% in those 60 to 70 years old, 25–30% in those 70–80 years old, and increases exponentially to more than 50% in persons aged 80–90 years [57].

Another major caveat is that a positive amyloid scan can also be seen not only in AD, but also in other medical conditions. For example, amyloid PET is frequently positive in DLB [58]. Nevertheless, [18F]FDG scans can play a role in identifying the 'cingulate island sign' (CIS), which is present in DLB and demonstrates increased glucose metabolism in the posterior cingulate cortex [59,60]. The CIS is highly specific for DLB (97–100%) but with lower sensitivity (62–86%) [60]. The sensitivity of detecting DLB by neuroimaging can be improved by presynaptic dopaminergic imaging using [123I]FP-CIT (DaTSCAN, GE Healthcare), which can give a pooled sensitivity of 86.5% (95% CI: 72–94.1%), but with relatively lower specificity of 93.6% (95% CI: 88.5–96.6%) [61]. Conversely, amyloid PET scans may, in certain instances, underestimate the brain amyloid plaque burden, especially in the setting of low cerebrospinal fluid (CSF) $A\beta_{42}$ levels and mild NCD of the AD type [62]. In cases of FTD, which has a similar insidious onset as AD but with predominantly language and behavioral abnormalities, [18F]FDG PET may detect hypometabolism more frequent in the frontal, anterior cingulate, and anterior temporal regions, as opposed to the temporo-parietal and posterior cingulate regions in AD [63]. Although there can be some overlapping areas that demonstrate [18F]FDG, PET amyloid scans often can differentiate FTD from AD as these cases demonstrate significantly lower amyloid uptake in frontal, temporo-parietal, and occipital lobes as well as in the putamen [64].

11. Conclusion

The aim of performing imaging scans in AD is to non-invasively aid in the diagnosis and provide objective confirmatory evidence of the cause of the neurocognitive deficit. This also aids the management of cognitive impairment, which includes prophylactic planning to anticipate future requirements of the patient. Overall, at present, PET amyloid imaging may promise a beneficial role to diagnose AD in inconclusive cases; however, there is an inherent limitation namely in its cost effectiveness and practical concerns for its execution due to many variations in protocols and cutoff values for interpretation of results.

12. Key Points

- $A\beta$ deposition can be accurately detected by PET amyloid scans.
- AD subjects will usually have a positive amyloid scan.
- Caution needs to be exercised during interpretation and reporting of scan results, as positive amyloid scans can be seen in cognitively normal older adults, AD, and other subtypes of dementia such as DLB.
- The degree of amyloid deposition does not correlate with the severity of AD.
- Severity of amyloid deposition in young subjects (with increased genetic susceptibility) may be a prognostic factor for the development of early onset AD among them.
- Amyloid PET qualitative evaluation of cerebral amyloid presence can be made by binary visual assessment, with loss of grey white matter differentiation denoting a positive scan.
- Quantification of $A\beta$ can be made using the whole cerebellum, cerebellar grey matter, and other regions of low to nil physiological amyloid deposition, as a reference point to calculate the standardised uptake value ratio (SUVr), using the assumption that these regions are usually spared in AD.

13. Recommendation

Future works should include recommendations for newer imaging radioligands, improved automated quantification of amyloid imaging, newer techniques for improved specificity in detecting subjects with Aβ deposition, and prognostication of at risk older adults for the possibility of developing Alzheimer's disease.

Author Contributions: S.S. and S.V. conceptualized this project. S.S. completed the original draft and M.-A.D. reviewed and edited the material. The entire project was done under S.V.'s supervision.

Funding: S.S. and M.-A.D. were both sponsored by the International Atomic Energy Agency (IAEA). S.S. received a scholarship for a Fellowship in Nuclear Medicine and focused on PET/CT and the IAEA made possible the collaboration with the Royal Liverpool and Broadgreen University Hospitals NHS Trusts, (RLBUHT) Liverpool, UK. M.-A.D. received a scholarship for a Fellowship in General Nuclear Medicine and the IAEA made possible the collaboration with the Royal Liverpool and Broadgreen University Hospitals NHS Trusts, (RLBUHT) Liverpool, UK.

Acknowledgments: We would like to express our gratitude to the Nuclear Medicine Unit of the Royal Liverpool and Broadgreen University Hospitals NHS Trusts, (RLBUHT) Liverpool, UK for granting permission to use anonymised images from the database. We also thank Mr. Ian Hufton, Principle Physicist in Nuclear Medicine, RLBUHT, Liverpool, UK for his assistance in image retrieval from the hospital achieving system.

Conflicts of Interest: The authors declare no conflict of interest.

References

1. Suppiah, S.; Ching, S.M.; Nordin, A.J.; Vinjamuri, S. The role of PET/CT amyloid Imaging compared with Tc99m-HMPAO-SPECT imaging for diagnosing Alzheimer's disease. *Med. J. Malays.* **2018**, *73*, 141–146.

2. Dhikav, V.; Sethi, M.; Anand, K.S. Medial temporal lobe atrophy in Alzheimer's disease/mild cognitive impairment with depression. *Bri. J. Radiol.* **2014**, *87*, 20140150. [CrossRef] [PubMed]

3. Suppiah, S.; Andi Asri, A.A.; Ahmad Saad, F.F.; Hassan, H.A.; Mohtarrudin, N.; Chang, W.L.; Mahmud, R.; Nordin, A.J. One stop centre staging by contrast-enhanced 18F-FDG PET/CT in preoperative assessment of ovarian cancer and proposed diagnostic imaging algorithm: A single centre experience in Malaysia. *MJMHS* **2017**, *13*, 29–37.

4. Ng, S.; Villemagne, V.L.; Berlangieri, S.; Lee, S.T.; Cherk, M.; Gong, S.J.; Ackermann, U.; Saunder, T.; Tochon-Danguy, H.; Jones, G.; et al. Visual Assessment Versus Quantitative Assessment of 11C-PIB PET and 18F-FDG PET for Detection of Alzheimer's Disease. *J. Nucl. Med.* **2007**, *48*, 547–552. [CrossRef] [PubMed]

5. Morris, J.C.; Price, J.L. Pathologic correlates of nondemented aging, mild cognitive impairment, and early-stage Alzheimer's disease. *J. Mol. Neurosci.* **2001**, *17*, 101–118. [CrossRef]

6. Anand, K.; Sabbagh, M. Amyloid Imaging: Poised for Integration into Medical Practice. *Neurotherapeutics* **2017**, *14*, 54–61. [CrossRef]

7. Degenhardt, E.K.; Witte, M.M.; Case, M.G.; Yu, P.; Henley, D.B.; Hochstetler, H.M.; D'Souza, D.N.; Trzepacz, P.T. Florbetapir F18 PET Amyloid Neuroimaging and Characteristics in Patients with Mild and Moderate Alzheimer Dementia. *Psychosomatics* **2016**, *57*, 208–216. [CrossRef]

8. Daerr, S.; Brendel, M.; Zach, C.; Mille, E.; Schilling, D.; Zacherl, M.J.; Bürger, K.; Danek, A.; Pogarell, O.; Schildan, A.; et al. Evaluation of early-phase [(18)F]-florbetaben PET acquisition in clinical routine cases. *NeuroImage Clin.* **2016**, *14*, 77–86. [CrossRef]

9. Lowe, V.J.; Lundt, E.; Knopman, D.; Senjem, M.L.; Gunter, J.L.; Schwarz, C.G.; Bradley, J.K.; Clifford, R.J.; Ronald, C.P. Comparison of [18F]Flutemetamol and [11C]Pittsburgh Compound-B in cognitively normal young, cognitively normal elderly, and Alzheimer's disease dementia individuals. *NeuroImage Clin.* **2017**, *16*, 295–302. [CrossRef]

10. Salloway, S.; Gamez, J.E.; Singh, U.; Sadowsky, C.H.; Villena, T.; Sabbagh, M.N.; Thomas, G.B.; Ranjan, D.; Adam, S.F.; Kirk, A.F.; et al. Performance of [(18)F]flutemetamol amyloid imaging against the neuritic plaque component of CERAD and the current (2012) NIA-AA recommendations for the neuropathologic diagnosis of Alzheimer's disease. *Alzheimers Dement.* **2017**, *9*, 25–34. [CrossRef]

11. Dukart, J.; Mueller, K.; Horstmann, A.; Vogt, B.; Frisch, S.; Barthel, H.; Becker, G.; Möller, H.E.; Villringer, A.; Sabri, O.; et al. Differential effects of global and cerebellar normalization on detection and differentiation of dementia in FDG-PET studies. *NeuroImage* **2010**, *49*, 1490–1495. [CrossRef] [PubMed]

12. Azmi, N.H.M.; Suppiah, S.; Liong, C.W.; Noor, N.M.; Said, S.M.; Hanafi, M.H.; Chalermrat, K.; Fathinul, F.A.S.; Sobhan, V. Reliability of standardized uptake value normalized to lean body mass using the liver as a reference organ, in contrast-enhanced 18F-FDG PET/CT imaging. *Radiat. Phys. Chem.* **2018**, *147*, 35–39. [CrossRef]

13. Cohen, A.D.; Klunk, W.E. Early detection of Alzheimer's disease using PiB and FDG PET. *Neurobiol. Dis.* **2014**, *72*, 117–122. [CrossRef] [PubMed]

14. Altmann, A.; Ng, B.; Greicius, M.D.; Landau, S.M.; Jagust, W.J. Regional brain hypometabolism is unrelated to regional amyloid plaque burden. *Brain* **2015**, *138*, 3734–3746. [CrossRef]

15. Cipriani, G.; Dolciotti, C.; Picchi, L.; Bonuccelli, U. Alzheimer and his disease: A brief history. *Neurol. Sci.* **2011**, *32*, 275–279. [CrossRef]

16. Prince, M.; Bryce, R.; Albanese, E.; Wimo, A.; Ribeiro, W.; Ferri, C.P. The global prevalence of dementia: A systematic review and metaanalysis. *Alzheimers Dement.* **2013**, *9*, 63–75.e62. [CrossRef]

17. American Psychiatric Association. *Diagnostic and Statistical Manual of Mental Disorders*, 5th ed.; American Psychiatric Publishing: Arlington, VA, USA, 2013; p. 947.

18. Trzepacz, P.T.; Hochstetler, H.; Wang, S.; Walker, B.; Saykin, A.J. Relationship between the Montreal Cognitive Assessment and Mini-mental State Examination for assessment of mild cognitive impairment in older adults. *BMC Geriatr.* **2015**, *15*, 107. [CrossRef]

19. McKhann, G.; Drachman, D.; Folstein, M.; Katzman, R.; Price, D.; Stadlan, E.M. Clinical diagnosis of Alzheimer's disease: Report of the NINCDS-ADRDA Work Group under the auspices of Department of Health and Human Services Task Force on Alzheimer's Disease. *Neurology* **1984**, *34*, 939–944. [CrossRef]

20. Knopman, D.S.; DeKosky, S.T.; Cummings, J.L.; Chui, H.; Corey-Bloom, J.; Relkin, N.; Small, G.W.; Miller, B.; Stevens, J.C. Practice parameter: diagnosis of dementia (an evidence-based review). Report of the Quality Standards Subcommittee of the American Academy of Neurology. *Neurology* **2001**, *56*, 1143–1153. [CrossRef]

21. McKhann, G.M.; Knopman, D.S.; Chertkow, H.; Hyman, B.T.; Jack, C.R.; Kawas, C.H.; Klunk, W.E.; Koroshetz, W.J.; Manly, J.J.; Mayeux, R.; et al. The diagnosis of dementia due to Alzheimer's disease: Recommendations from the National Institute on Aging-Alzheimer's Association workgroups on diagnostic guidelines for Alzheimer's disease. *Alzheimers Dement.* **2011**, *7*, 263–269. [CrossRef]

22. Neary, D.; Snowden, J.; Mann, D. Frontotemporal dementia. *Lancet Neurol.* **2005**, *4*, 771–780. [CrossRef]

23. Dubois, B.; Feldman, H.H.; Jacova, C.; Hampel, H.; Molinuevo, J.L.; Blennow, K.; DeKosky, S.T.; Gauthier, S.; Selkoe, D.; Bateman, R.; et al. Advancing research diagnostic criteria for Alzheimer's disease: the IWG-2 criteria. *Lancet Neurol.* **2014**, *13*, 614–629. [CrossRef]

24. Higashi, T.; Nishii, R.; Kagawa, S.; Kishibe, Y.; Takahashi, M.; Okina, T.; Suzuki, N.; Hasegawa, H.; Nagahama, Y.; Ishizu, K.; et al. 18 F-FPYBF-2, a new F-18-labelled amyloid imaging PET tracer: First experience in 61 volunteers and 55 patients with dementia. *Ann. Nucl. Med.* **2018**, *32*, 206–216. [CrossRef] [PubMed]

25. Klunk, W.E.; Engler, H.; Nordberg, A.; Wang, Y.; Blomqvist, G.; Holt, D.P.; Bergström, M.; Savitcheva, I.; Huang, G.F.; Estrada, S.; et al. Imaging brain amyloid in Alzheimer's disease with Pittsburgh Compound-B. *Ann. Neurol.* **2004**, *55*, 306–319. [CrossRef] [PubMed]

26. Rowe, C.C.; Ng, S.; Ackermann, U.; Gong, S.J.; Pike, K.; Savage, G.; Cowie, T.F.; Dickinson, K.L.; Maruff, P.; Darby, D.; et al. Imaging beta-amyloid burden in aging and dementia. *Neurology* **2007**, *68*, 1718–1725. [CrossRef] [PubMed]

27. Jack, C.R., Jr.; Wiste, H.J.; Weigand, S.D.; Knopman, D.S.; Lowe, V.; Vemuri, P.; Mielke, M.M.; Jones, D.T.; Senjem, M.L.; Gunter, J.L.; et al. Amyloid-first and neurodegeneration-first profiles characterize incident amyloid PET positivity. *Neurology* **2013**, *81*, 1732–1740. [CrossRef] [PubMed]

28. Clark, C.M.; Schneider, J.A.; Bedell, B.J.; Beach, T.G.; Bilker, W.B.; Mintun, M.A.; Pontecorvo, M.J.; Hefti, F.; Carpenter, A.P.; Flitter, M.L.; et al. Use of florbetapir-PET for imaging beta-amyloid pathology. *JAMA* **2011**, *305*, 275–283. [CrossRef]

29. Wong, D.F.; Rosenberg, P.B.; Zhou, Y.; Kumar, A.; Raymont, V.; Ravert, H.T.; Dannals, R.F.; Nandi, A.; Brasić, J.R.; Ye, W.; et al. In vivo imaging of amyloid deposition in Alzheimer disease using the radioligand ^{18}F-AV-45 (florbetapir F 18). *J. Nucl. Med.* **2010**, *51*, 913–920. [CrossRef]

30. Filippi, L.; Chiaravalloti, A.; Bagni, O.; Schillaci, O. (18)F-labeled radiopharmaceuticals for the molecular neuroimaging of amyloid plaques in Alzheimer's disease. *Am. J. Nucl. Med. Mol. Imaging* **2018**, *8*, 268–281.

31. Rodrigue, K.M.; Rieck, J.R.; Kennedy, K.M.; Devous, M.D., Sr.; Diaz-Arrastia, R.; Park, D.C. Risk factors for β-amyloid deposition in healthy aging: vascular and genetic effects. *JAMA Neurol.* **2013**, *70*, 600–606. [CrossRef]

32. Villemagne, V.L.; Mulligan, R.S.; Pejoska, S.; Ong, K.; Jones, G.; O'Keefe, G.; Chan, J.G.; Young, K.; Tochon-Danguy, H.; Masters, C.L.; et al. Comparison of 11C-PiB and 18F-florbetaben for Abeta imaging in ageing and Alzheimer's disease. *Eur. J. Nucl. Med. Mol. Imaging* **2012**, *39*, 983–989. [CrossRef]

33. Ataka, S.; Takeda, A.; Mino, T.; Yamakawa, Y.; Yamamoto, K.; Tsutada, T.; Kawabe, J.; Wada, Y.; Shiomi, S.; Watanabe, Y.; et al. Comparison of [18F] Flutemetamol and [11C] PIB PET images. *Alzheimers Dement.* **2014**, *10*, P21. [CrossRef]

34. Rabinovici, G.D.; Schonhaut, D.; Baker, S.; Lazaris, A.; Ossenkoppele, R.; Lockhart, S.; Schöll, M.; Schwimmer, H.; Vogel, J.; Ayakta, N.; et al. Tau PET with [^{18}F]AV1451 in non-alzheimer's disease neurodegenerative syndromes. *Alzheimers Dement.* **2015**, *11*, P107–P109. [CrossRef]

35. Siderowf, A.; Pontecorvo, M.J.; Shill, H.A.; Mintun, M.A.; Arora, A.; Joshi, A.D.; Lu, M.; Adler, C.H.; Galasko, D.; Liebsack, C.; et al. PET imaging of amyloid with Florbetapir F18 and PET imaging of dopamine degeneration with 18F-AV-133 (florbenazine) in patients with Alzheimer's disease and Lewy body disorders. *BMC Neurol.* **2014**, *14*, 79. [CrossRef] [PubMed]

36. Sadigh-Eteghad, S.; Sabermarouf, B.; Majdi, A.; Talebi, M.; Farhoudi, M.; Mahmoudi, J. Amyloid-beta: A crucial factor in Alzheimer's disease. *Med. Princ. Pract.* **2015**, *24*, 1–10. [CrossRef] [PubMed]

37. Mormino, E.C.; Kluth, J.T.; Madison, C.M.; Rabinovici, G.D.; Baker, S.L.; Miller, B.L.; Koeppe, R.A.; Mathis, C.A.; Weiner, M.W.; Jagust, W.J. Episodic memory loss is related to hippocampal-mediated beta-amyloid deposition in elderly subjects. *Brain* **2009**, *132 Pt 5*, 1310–1323. [CrossRef]

38. Hardy, J.; Selkoe, D.J. The amyloid hypothesis of Alzheimer's disease: progress and problems on the road to therapeutics. *Science* **2002**, *297*, 353–356. [CrossRef]

39. Bateman, R.J.; Xiong, C.; Benzinger, T.L.; Fagan, A.M.; Goate, A.; Fox, N.C.; Marcus, D.S.; Cairns, N.J.; Xie, X.; Blazey, T.M.; et al. Clinical and biomarker changes in dominantly inherited Alzheimer's disease. *N. Engl. J. Med.* **2012**, *367*, 795–804. [CrossRef]

40. Chiang, G.C.; Mao, X.; Kang, G.; Chang, E.; Pandya, S.; Vallabhajosula, S.; Isaacson, R.; Ravdin, L.D. Relationships among cortical glutathione levels, brain amyloidosis, and memory in healthy older adults investigated in vivo with 1H-MRS and Pittsburgh compound-B PET. *Am. J. Neuroradiol.* **2017**, *38*, 1130–1137. [CrossRef]

41. Chiaravalloti, A.; Castellano, A.E.; Ricci, M.; Barbagallo, G.; Sannino, P.; Ursini, F.; Karalis, G.; Schillaci, O. Coupled Imaging with [18F]FBB and [18F]FDG in AD Subjects Show a Selective Association Between Amyloid Burden and Cortical Dysfunction in the Brain. *Mol. Imaging Biol.* **2018**, *20*, 659–666. [CrossRef]

42. Ciarmiello, A.; Tartaglione, A.; Giovannini, E.; Riondato, M.; Giovacchini, G.; Ferrando, O.; De Biasi, M.; Passera, C.; Carabelli, E.; Mannironi, A.; et al. Amyloid burden identifies neuropsychological phenotypes at increased risk of progression to Alzheimer's disease in mild cognitive impairment patients. *Eur. J. Nucl. Med. Mol. Imaging* **2019**, *46*, 288–296. [CrossRef] [PubMed]

43. Miki, T.; Shimada, H.; Kim, J.S.; Yamamoto, Y.; Sugino, M.; Kowa, H.; Heurling, K.; Zanette, M.; Sherwin, P.F.; Senda, M. Brain uptake and safety of Flutemetamol F 18 injection in Japanese subjects with probable Alzheimer's disease, subjects with amnestic mild cognitive impairment and healthy volunteers. *Ann. Nucl. Med.* **2017**, *31*, 260–272. [CrossRef] [PubMed]

44. Pothier, K.; Saint-Aubert, L.; Hooper, C.; Delrieu, J.; Payoux, P.; de Souto Barreto, P.; Vellas, B. MAPT/DSA Study Group. Cognitive changes of older adults with an equivocal amyloid load. *J. Neurol.* **2019**, *266*, 835–843. [CrossRef] [PubMed]

45. Johnson, K.A.; Minoshima, S.; Bohnen, N.I.; Donohoe, K.J.; Foster, N.L.; Herscovitch, P.; Karlawish, J.H.; Rowe, C.C.; Carrillo, M.C.; Hartley, D.M.; et al. Appropriate use criteria for amyloid PET: A report of the Amyloid Imaging Task Force, the Society of Nuclear Medicine and Molecular Imaging, and the Alzheimer's Association. *Alzheimers Dement.* **2013**, *9*, e-1-16. [CrossRef] [PubMed]

46. Alongi, P.; Sardina, D.S.; Coppola, R.; Scalisi, S.; Puglisi, V.; Arnone, A.; Raimondo, G.D.; Munerati, E.; Alaimo, V.; Midiri, F.; et al. 18F-Florbetaben PET/CT to Assess Alzheimer's Disease: A new Analysis Method for Regional Amyloid Quantification. *J. Neuroimaging* **2019**, *3*, 383–393. [CrossRef]

47. Bouter, C.; Vogelgsang, J.; Wiltfang, J. Comparison between amyloid-PET and CSF amyloid-β biomarkers in a clinical cohort with memory deficits. *Clin. Chim. Acta* **2019**, *492*, 62–68. [CrossRef]

48. Frings, L.; Hellwig, S.; Bormann, T.; Spehl, T.S.; Buchert, R.; Meyer, P.T. Amyloid load but not regional glucose metabolism predicts conversion to Alzheimer's dementia in a memory clinic population. *Eur. J. Nucl. Med. Mol. Imaging* **2018**, *45*, 1442–1448. [CrossRef]

49. Kim, S.E.; Woo, S.; Kim, S.W.; Chin, J.; Kim, H.J.; Lee, B.I.; Park, J.; Park, K.W.; Kang, D.Y.; Noh, Y.; et al. A nomogram for predicting amyloid PET positivity in amnestic mild cognitive impairment. *J. Alzheimers Dis.* **2018**, *66*, 681–691. [CrossRef]

50. Schmidt, M.E.; Chiao, P.; Klein, G.; Matthews, D.; Thurfjell, L.; Cole, P.E.; Margolin, R.; Landau, S.; Foster, N.L.; Mason, N.S.; et al. The influence of biological and technical factors on quantitative analysis of amyloid PET: Points to consider and recommendations for controlling variability in longitudinal data. *Alzheimers Dement.* **2015**, *11*, 1050–1068. [CrossRef]

51. Newberg, A.B.; Arnold, S.E.; Wintering, N.; Rovner, B.W.; Alavi, A. Initial clinical comparison of 18F-florbetapir and 18F-FDG PET in patients with Alzheimer disease and controls. *J. Nucl Med.* **2012**, *53*, 902–907. [CrossRef]

52. La Joie, R.; Perrotin, A.; Barre, L.; Hommet, C.; Mezenge, F.; Ibazizene, M.; Camus, V.; Abbas, A.; Landeau, B.; Guilloteau, D.; et al. Region-specific hierarchy between atrophy, hypometabolism, and beta-amyloid (Abeta) load in Alzheimer's disease dementia. *J. Neurosci.* **2012**, *32*, 16265–16273. [CrossRef] [PubMed]

53. Pfefferbaum, A.; Chanraud, S.; Pitel, A.-L.; Müller-Oehring, E.; Shankaranarayanan, A.; Alsop, D.C.; Rohlfing, T.; Sullivan, E.V. Cerebral blood flow in posterior cortical nodes of the default mode network decreases with task engagement but remains higher than in most brain regions. *Cereb. Cortex* **2011**, *21*, 233–244. [CrossRef] [PubMed]

54. Fleisher, A.S.; Chen, K.; Liu, X.; Roontiva, A.; Thiyyagura, P.; Ayutyanont, N.; Joshi, A.D.; Clark, C.M.; Mintun, M.A.; Pontecorvo, M.J.; et al. Using positron emission tomography and florbetapir F18 to image cortical amyloid in patients with mild cognitive impairment or dementia due to Alzheimer disease. *Arch. Neurol.* **2011**, *68*, 1404–1411. [CrossRef] [PubMed]

55. Camus, V.; Payoux, P.; Barré, L.; Desgranges, B.; Voisin, T.; Tauber, C.; La Joie, R.; Tafani, M.; Hommet, C.; Chételat, G.; et al. Using PET with 18F-AV-45 (florbetapir) to quantify brain amyloid load in a clinical environment. *Europ. J. Nucl. Medi. Mol. Imaging* **2012**, *39*, 621–631. [CrossRef] [PubMed]

56. Klupp, E.; Grimmer, T.; Tahmasian, M.; Sorg, C.; Yakushev, I.; Yousefi, B.H.; Drzezga, A.; Förster, S. Prefrontal hypometabolism in Alzheimer disease is related to longitudinal amyloid accumulation in remote brain regions. *J. Nucl. Med.* **2015**, *56*, 399–404. [CrossRef] [PubMed]

57. Marcus, C.; Mena, E.; Subramaniam, R.M. Brain PET in the diagnosis of Alzheimer's disease. *Clin. Nucl. Med.* **2014**, *39*, e413–e426. [CrossRef]

58. Kantarci, K.; Yang, C.; Schneider, J.A.; Senjem, M.L.; Reyes, D.A.; Lowe, V.J.; Barnes, L.L.; Aggarwal, N.T.; Bennett, D.A.; Smith, G.E.; et al. Antemortem amyloid imaging and β-amyloid pathology in a case with dementia with Lewy bodies. *Neurobiol. Aging* **2012**, *33*, 878–885. [CrossRef]

59. Iizuka, T.; Kameyama, M. Cingulate island sign on FDG-PET is associated with medial temporal lobe atrophy in dementia with Lewy bodies. *Ann. Nucl. Med.* **2016**, *30*, 421–429. [CrossRef]

60. Lim, S.M.; Katsifis, A.; Villemagne, V.L.; Best, R.; Jones, G.; Saling, M.; Bradshaw, J.; Merory, J.; Woodward, M.; Hopwood, M.; et al. The 18F-FDG PET cingulate island sign and comparison to 123I-beta-CIT SPECT for diagnosis of dementia with Lewy bodies. *J. Nucl. Med.* **2009**, *50*, 1638–1645. [CrossRef]

61. Papathanasiou, N.D.; Boutsiadis, A.; Dickson, J.; Bomanji, J.B. Diagnostic accuracy of 123I-FP-CIT (DaTSCAN) in dementia with Lewy bodies: A meta-analysis of published studies. *Parkinsonism Relat. Disord.* **2012**, *18*, 225–229. [CrossRef]

62. Lewczuk, P.; Matzen, A.; Blennow, K.; Parnetti, L.; Molinuevo, J.L.; Eusebi, P.; Kornhuber, J.; Morris, J.C.; Fagan, A.M. Cerebrospinal Fluid Abeta42/40 Corresponds Better than Abeta42 to Amyloid PET in Alzheimer's Disease. *J. Alzheimers Dis.* **2017**, *55*, 813–822. [CrossRef] [PubMed]

63. Foster, N.L.; Heidebrink, J.L.; Clark, C.M.; Jagust, W.J.; Arnold, S.E.; Barbas, N.R.; DeCarli, C.S.; Turner, R.S.; Koeppe, R.A.; Higdon, R.; et al. FDG-PET improves accuracy in distinguishing frontotemporal dementia and Alzheimer's disease. *Brain* **2007**, *130*, 2616–2635. [CrossRef] [PubMed]

64. Engler, H.; Santillo, A.F.; Wang, S.X.; Lindau, M.; Savitcheva, I.; Nordberg, A.; Lannfelt, L.; Långström, B.; Kilander, L. In vivo amyloid imaging with PET in frontotemporal dementia. *Eur. J. Nucl. Med. Mol. Imaging* **2008**, *35*, 100–106. [CrossRef] [PubMed]

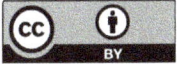

diagnostics

MDPI

Article

Lower CSF Amyloid-Beta$_{1-42}$ Predicts a Higher Mortality Rate in Frontotemporal Dementia

Daniela Vieira [1,†], João Durães [1,†], Inês Baldeiras [1,2,3], Beatriz Santiago [1], Diana Duro [1], Marisa Lima [1], Maria João Leitão [1,3], Miguel Tábuas-Pereira [1,*,‡] and Isabel Santana [1,2,3,‡]

[1] Neurology Department, Centro Hospitalar e Universitário de Coimbra, 3000-045 Coimbra, Portugal;
    danielacgvieira@gmail.com (D.V.); duraes.jlo@gmail.com (J.D.); ines.baldeiras@sapo.pt (I.B.);
    hbmcsantiago@hotmail.com (B.S.); diana.duro@gmail.com (D.D.); marisalima5@hotmail.com (M.L.);
    jajao86@gmail.com (M.J.L.); isabeljsantana@gmail.com (I.S.)
[2] Faculty of Medicine, University of Coimbra, 3000-070 Coimbra, Portugal
[3] Center for Neuroscience and Cell Biology, University of Coimbra, 3000-070 Coimbra, Portugal
*   Correspondence: miguelatcp@gmail.com
†   These authors contributed equally to this work.
‡   These authors contributed equally to this work.

Received: 30 September 2019; Accepted: 22 October 2019; Published: 25 October 2019

Abstract: Frontotemporal lobar degeneration, the neuropathological substrate of frontotemporal dementia (FTD), is characterized by the deposition of protein aggregates, including tau. Evidence has shown concomitant amyloid pathology in some of these patients, which seems to contribute to a more aggressive disease. Our aim was to evaluate cerebrospinal fluid (CSF) amyloid-beta as a predictor of the mortality of FTD patients. We included 99 patients diagnosed with FTD—both behavioral and language variants—with no associated motor neuron disease, from whom a CSF sample was collected. These patients were followed prospectively in our center, and demographic and clinical data were obtained. The survival analysis was carried through a Cox regression model. Patients who died during follow up had a significantly lower CSF amyloid-beta$_{1-42}$ than those who did not. The survival analysis demonstrated that an increased death rate was associated with a lower CSF amyloid-beta$_{1-42}$ (HR = 0.999, 95% CI = [0.997, 1.000], $p = 0.049$). Neither demographic nor clinical variables, nor CSF total tau or p-tau were significantly associated with this endpoint. These results suggest that amyloid deposition in FTD patients may be associated with a higher mortality.

Keywords: frontotemporal dementia; amyloid; cerebrospinal fluid; mortality

1. Introduction

Frontotemporal dementia (FTD) is a progressive neurodegenerative clinical syndrome, characterized by changes in behavior, executive function, and language. It is generally classified in three clinical variants: behavioral-variant FTD, non-fluent variant primary progressive aphasia, and semantic-variant primary progressive aphasia.

The neuropathological substrate, frontotemporal lobar degeneration, is characterized by neuronal loss, gliosis, and microvacuolar changes of the frontal lobes, anterior temporal lobes, anterior cingulate cortex, and insular cortex. Different subtypes are associated with abnormal deposition of different proteins, namely microtubule-associated protein tau, the TAR DNA-binding protein with molecular weight 43 kDa, or the fused-in-sarcoma protein [1].

On the contrary, amyloid-beta$_{1-42}$ deposition is a hallmark of Alzheimer's disease (AD). However, patients with FTD may have superimposed amyloid pathology [2]. Recently, amyloid-beta plaques have been found to facilitate the aggregation of tau [3] in AD models. Interestingly, in FTD patients with pathogenic mutations, amyloid has also been shown to be associated with a worse performance in several cognitive tests [4]. Additionally, CSF amyloid has been shown to be associated with higher volumetric loss in sporadic FTD patients [5].

We aimed to evaluate the value of cerebrospinal (CSF) amyloid-beta$_{1-42}$ as a predictor of mortality in FTD patients.

2. Materials and Methods

2.1. Patient Selection

Our study included patients that fulfilled the current diagnostic criteria for behavioral variant of FTD [6] or language variants [7] with probable FTD-associated pathology, recruited at the Dementia Outpatient Clinic of the Centro Hospitalar e Universitário de Coimbra (Portugal). Defined inclusion criteria mandated a full neuropsychological evaluation and CSF biomarkers analysis. Patients who presented with motor neuron disorder at any point along the follow-up period were excluded. For the survival analysis, we considered the interval between the time of the lumbar puncture (LP)—baseline—and the time of death.

These patients are part of a prospectively evaluated cohort at our center. For the purpose of this study, we collected demographical data (age of onset, age at LP, gender, family history, and years of formal education), vascular risk factors at the time of the LP (history of diabetes, high blood pressure, dyslipidemia, atrial fibrillation, obesity, heart failure, coronary artery disease, heart valve disease, alcohol abuse, smoking, sleep obstructive apnea, and stroke), Mini-Mental State Examination (MMSE), and Clinical Dementia Rating (CDR) score at the time of LP.

The study was conducted according to the revised Declaration of Helsinki and Good Clinical Practice guidelines. Informed consent was given by all study participants or their legal next of kin. This project was approved by the ethics committee of our center, with the code HUC-43-09, prior to the beginning of the study.

2.2. CSF Biomarkers

CSF samples were collected as part of the routine clinical diagnostic protocol. Pre-analytical and analytical procedures were done in accordance with the Alzheimer's Association guidelines for CSF biomarker determination [8]. CSF samples were collected in sterile polypropylene tubes, immediately centrifuged at 1800 g for 10 min at 4 °C, aliquoted into polypropylene tubes and stored at −80 °C until analysis. CSF Aβ42, T-tau, and P-tau were measured separately by commercially available sandwich ELISA kits (Innotest, Fujirebio, Belgium), as previously described [9,10]. External quality control of the assays was performed under the scope of the Alzheimer's Association Quality Control Program for CSF Biomarkers [8].

2.3. Statistical Analysis

Statistical analysis was performed using the SPSS statistical software (version 20.0; SPSS Inc., Chicago, IL, USA). Categorical data are presented as frequency (percentage) and were compared using χ^2-test. Ordinal or discrete risk factors are represented using median values and compared using the Mann−Whitney U test. Comparison of the measured variables between the different groups was performed using a Student's t-test or γ^2 test.

To assess for independent associations with death, a Cox regression was performed, adjusted for the collected data: age at onset, age at LP, CDR at the time of LP, CSF biomarkers, and behavioral versus language variants. Vascular risk factors with significant differences between patients who died during follow up and those who did not were also included. All the assumptions of these models were verified. Statistical significance was set at $\alpha = 0.05$.

3. Results

We included 116 patients. Eight patients were lost to follow-up. Nine were excluded for having developed a motor neuron disorder. Finally, we included 99 patients, with a mean follow-up duration of 5.0 (±2.8) years. Mean age of onset was 61.4 (±9.3) years old. Male patients composed 46.9% of the cohort. Median education was 4.0 (IQR = 5.0) years. From the whole sample, 32 (33.3%) patients died during the follow-up period (average follow-up period for this subset of 5.0 ± 3.0 years). Table 1 presents the comparison of patients who died and those who did not during the follow-up period in terms of the studied variables. Vascular risk factors prevalence and comparison may be found in Supplementary Table S1.

Table 1. Comparison of the two groups in terms of the studied variables.

Variable	Mean Values for the Whole Sample	Mean Values for Patients Who Died during Follow-Up	Mean Values For Patients Who Did Not Die during Follow-Up	p
Sex (% male)	46.9	50.0	45.3	0.664
Variant (% behavioral variant)	85.4	87.5	84.4	0.683
Family history (% positive)	30.2	28.1	31.3	0.753
Age of onset (years)	61.4 (±9.3)	61.1 (±9.8)	61.5 (±9.2)	0.831
Age at LP (years)	63.5 (±9.6)	62.9 (±10.1)	63.9 (9.6)	0.664
Education (years) (median, IQR)	4.0 (IQR = 5.0)	4.0 (IQR = 5.0)	4.0 (IQR = 5.0)	0.791
MMSE at LP	21.1 (±6.8)	20.0 (±7.1)	21.6 (±6.4)	0.271
CDR at LP (median, IQR)	1.0 (IQR = 1.0)	1.0 (IQR = 1.0)	1.0 (IQR = 0.0)	0.016
Follow-up (years)	5.0 (±2.8)	4.5 (±2.6)	5.0 (±3.0)	0.468
CSF amyloid-beta$_{1-42}$ (pg/mL)	677.5 (±301.8)	532.7 (±306.0)	731.8 (±279.2)	0.002
CSF tau (pg/mL)	338.9 (±371.1)	277.6 (±166.5)	365.2 (±429.4)	0.286
CSF phosphorylated-tau (pg/mL)	41.4 (±38.4)	34.8 (±16.2)	44.7 (±44.4)	0.223

LP: lumbar puncture. MMSE: Mini-Mental State Examination, CDR: Clinical Dementia Rating, CSF: Cerebrospinal Fluid.

In terms of vascular risk factors, patients who died during follow-up had a significant lower prevalence of high blood pressure (28.1% vs. 52.2%, p = 0.024), diabetes (6.3% vs. 23.9%, p = 0.033), and dyslipidemia (18.8% vs. 49.3%, p = 0.004). No significant differences were found in the other vascular risk factors (Supplementary Table S1).

In the univariate analysis, death was associated with CSF amyloid-beta$_{1-42}$ levels and CDR. In Cox regression (Table 2), the risk of death was associated with CSF amyloid-beta$_{1-42}$ levels (HR = 0.999, 95%CI = [0.997, 1.000], p = 0.049).

Table 2. Cox regression results of the variables associated with the death rate ($\gamma^2 = 18.799$, df = 10, $p = 0.043$, −2 log likelihood = 225.540).

Variable	HR	95% CI	p
Age of onset	0.951	0.807, 1.120	0.546
Age at lumbar puncture	1.097	0.933, 1.289	0.261
Behavioral variant	0.634	0.147, 2.736	0.542
CDR	1.692	0.983, 2.914	0.058
CSF Amyloid-beta$_{1-42}$	0.999	0.997, 1.000	0.049
CSF total tau	1.001	0.998, 1.004	0.514
CSF phosphorylated tau	0.985	0.956, 1.014	0.305
Diabetes	0.428	0.087, 2.118	0.298
High blood pressure	0.735	0.301. 1.794	0.499
Dyslipidemia	0.403	0.142, 1.147	0.089

HR: Hazard ratio; CI: Confidence interval; CSF: cerebrospinal fluid.

4. Discussion

We report a relatively large size sample of thoroughly studied frontotemporal dementia patients. We found a significant independent association between lower CSF amyloid-beta$_{1-42}$ levels and higher mortality.

There is a lack of good FTD diagnostic and prognostic biomarkers. Neurofilament light chain, total Tau [11], and phosphorylated-Tau/total-Tau ratio have been reported to have some clinical value [5,12–15]. Neurofilament light chain has also been shown to be correlated with disease severity, brain atrophy, annualized brain atrophy, and survival [16]. Additionally, some studies have shown that amyloid-positive patients perform significantly worse in cognitive tests [4]. Also, low baseline amyloid-beta$_{1-42}$ has been associated with faster radiographic change in bvFTD [5].

In our sample, amyloid-beta$_{1-42}$ has shown value as a marker of higher mortality rate (HR = 0.999, 95% CI = [0.997, 1.000], $p = 0.049$). If, on one hand, the clinical value of this association might be low, the biological link it represents may be of great importance in the understanding of the biological processes underlying this (and possibly other) conditions. In fact, it has been recently suggested that amyloid-beta plaques enhance tau-seeded pathologies by facilitating neuritic plaque tau aggregation [3]. This facilitation may happen through different mechanisms, such as the creation of a microenvironment that enhances the recruitment of tau into fibrils, but also by impairment of intracellular protein degradation [17].

This may be one explanation for these findings, but other hypotheses may be put forward, such as the occurrence of co-pathology (19.2% of the patients had reduced CSF amyloid-beta$_{1-42}$). However, the rather young age of these patients makes it less likely that Alzheimer's pathology may cause a great disease burden. On the other hand, it could be that, in the presence of concurring FTD-related pathology, a less advanced Alzheimer's pathology could cause a more severe dysfunction. There is evidence that extracellular tau regulates the production of amyloid-beta, by mediating neuronal hyperactivity [18]. The amyloid-beta$_{1-42}$ values could, therefore, be a reflection of a downstream impact of extracellular tau. In the absence of pathologic confirmation, misdiagnosis in a part of the sample is always a possibility. But these patients have been extensively studied and followed for several years. Moreover, one would expect that AD patients (who would have lower CSF amyloid-beta$_{1-42}$ values) would progress slower than the FTD patients [19], however, this is an inverse relationship of what we found.

One important consideration is concerning vascular risk factors, as there were some differences in their prevalence on univariate analysis. In fact, the patients who did not die during the follow-up have a higher prevalence of some of these risk factors (diabetes, high blood pressure, and dyslipidemia) than those who have died. This is in line with some previous studies [20]. This may mean that the patients with a more rapid course have other strong factors driving the progression (possibly genetic), rather than a more multifactorial disease in the group of patients who did not die. These results could also mean that some of the patients in the group of patients who did not die during follow-up may have vascular dementia rather than frontotemporal dementia, leading to a more slowly progressive disease.

The main limitation of our work is its retrospective nature, although the data were prospectively collected, the hypothesis may be biased. Additionally, we do not have pathological data, and, since frontotemporal dementia may be associated with different pathological patterns and deposition of different proteins, the association with CSF amyloid-beta$_{1-42}$ may be true only for one of these pathologies. However, the hard endpoint that we have measured (progression), and the moderate size of the sample, support the generalizability of these results.

5. Conclusions

Our results suggest that CSF amyloid-beta$_{1-42}$ may modulate mortality in frontotemporal dementia patients.

Supplementary Materials: The following are available online at http://www.mdpi.com/2075-4418/9/4/162/s1, Table S1: Comparison of the two groups in terms of vascular risk factors.

Author Contributions: Conceptualization—M.T.-P., D.V., J.D. and I.S.; methodology—I.B., B.S., D.D., M.L., M.J.L., I.S. and M.T.-P.; software—M.T.-P.; validation—M.T.-P., I.S.; formal analysis—all authors; investigation, all authors; writing—original draft preparation—D.V., M.T.-P. and J.D.; writing—review and editing—I.S., M.T.-P. and I.B.

Funding: This research received no external funding.

Conflicts of Interest: The authors declare no conflict of interest.

References

1. Bang, J.; Spina, S.; Miller, B.L. Frontotemporal dementia. *Lancet* **2015**, *386*, 1672–1682. [CrossRef]
2. Rohrer, J.D.; Lashley, T.; Schott, J.M.; Warren, J.E.; Mead, S.; Isaacs, A.M.; Beck, J.; Hardy, J.; de Silva, R.; Warrington, E.; et al. Clinical and neuroanatomical signatures of tissue pathology in frontotemporal lobar degeneration. *Brain A J. Neurol.* **2011**, *134*, 2565–2581. [CrossRef] [PubMed]
3. He, Z.; Guo, J.L.; McBride, J.D.; Narasimhan, S.; Kim, H.; Changolkar, L.; Zhang, B.; Gathagan, R.J.; Yue, C.; Dengler, C.; et al. Amyloid-beta plaques enhance Alzheimer's brain tau-seeded pathologies by facilitating neuritic plaque tau aggregation. *Nat. Med.* **2018**, *24*, 29–38. [CrossRef] [PubMed]
4. Naasan, G.; Rabinovici, G.D.; Ghosh, P.; Elofson, J.D.; Miller, B.L.; Coppola, G.; Karydas, A.; Fong, J.; Perry, D.; Lee, S.E.; et al. Amyloid in dementia associated with familial FTLD: Not an innocent bystander. *Neurocase* **2016**, *22*, 76–83. [CrossRef]
5. Ljubenkov, P.A.; Staffaroni, A.M.; Rojas, J.C.; Allen, I.E.; Wang, P.; Heuer, H.; Karydas, A.; Kornak, J.; Cobigo, Y.; Seeley, W.W.; et al. Cerebrospinal fluid biomarkers predict frontotemporal dementia trajectory. *Ann. Clin. Transl. Neurol.* **2018**, *5*, 1250–1263. [CrossRef]
6. Rascovsky, K.; Hodges, J.R.; Knopman, D.; Mendez, M.F.; Kramer, J.H.; Neuhaus, J.; van Swieten, J.C.; Seelaar, H.; Dopper, E.G.; Onyike, C.U.; et al. Sensitivity of revised diagnostic criteria for the behavioural variant of frontotemporal dementia. *Brain* **2011**, *134*, 2456–2477. [CrossRef] [PubMed]
7. Gorno-Tempini, M.L.; Hillis, A.E.; Weintraub, S.; Kertesz, A.; Mendez, M.; Cappa, S.F.; Ogar, J.M.; Rohrer, J.D.; Black, S.; Boeve, B.F.; et al. Classification of primary progressive aphasia and its variants. *Neurology* **2011**, *76*, 1006–1014. [CrossRef] [PubMed]
8. Mattsson, N.; Andreasson, U.; Persson, S.; Arai, H.; Batish, S.D.; Bernardini, S.; Bocchio-Chiavetto, L.; Blankenstein, M.A.; Carrillo, M.C.; Chalbot, S.; et al. The Alzheimer's Association external quality control program for cerebrospinal fluid biomarkers. *Alzheimer's Dement.* **2011**, *7*, 386–395. [CrossRef] [PubMed]
9. Baldeiras, I.E.; Ribeiro, M.H.; Pacheco, P.; Machado, A.; Santana, I.; Cunha, L.; Oliveira, C.R. Diagnostic value of CSF protein profile in a Portuguese population of sCJD patients. *J. Neurol.* **2009**, *256*, 1540–1550. [CrossRef] [PubMed]

10. Kapaki, E.; Kilidireas, K.; Paraskevas, G.P.; Michalopoulou, M.; Patsouris, E. Highly increased CSF tau protein and decreased beta-amyloid (1-42) in sporadic CJD: A discrimination from Alzheimer's disease? *J. Neurol. Neurosurg. Psychiatry* **2001**, *71*, 401–403. [CrossRef] [PubMed]

11. Borroni, B.; Benussi, A.; Cosseddu, M.; Archetti, S.; Padovani, A. Cerebrospinal fluid tau levels predict prognosis in non-inherited frontotemporal dementia. *Neuro.-Degener. Dis.* **2014**, *13*, 224–229. [CrossRef] [PubMed]

12. Meeter, L.H.H.; Vijverberg, E.G.; Del Campo, M.; Rozemuller, A.J.M.; Donker Kaat, L.; de Jong, F.J.; van der Flier, W.M.; Teunissen, C.E.; van Swieten, J.C.; Pijnenburg, Y.A.L. Clinical value of neurofilament and phospho-tau/tau ratio in the frontotemporal dementia spectrum. *Neurology* **2018**, *90*, e1231–e1239. [CrossRef] [PubMed]

13. Borroni, B.; Benussi, A.; Archetti, S.; Galimberti, D.; Parnetti, L.; Nacmias, B.; Sorbi, S.; Scarpini, E.; Padovani, A. Csf p-tau181/tau ratio as biomarker for TDP pathology in frontotemporal dementia. *Amyotroph. Lateral Scler. Front. Degener.* **2015**, *16*, 86–91. [CrossRef] [PubMed]

14. Hu, W.T.; Watts, K.; Grossman, M.; Glass, J.; Lah, J.J.; Hales, C.; Shelnutt, M.; Van Deerlin, V.; Trojanowski, J.Q.; Levey, A.I. Reduced CSF p-Tau181 to Tau ratio is a biomarker for FTLD-TDP. *Neurology* **2013**, *81*, 1945–1952. [CrossRef] [PubMed]

15. Pijnenburg, Y.A.; Verwey, N.A.; van der Flier, W.M.; Scheltens, P.; Teunissen, C.E. Discriminative and prognostic potential of cerebrospinal fluid phosphoTau/tau ratio and neurofilaments for frontotemporal dementia subtypes. *Alzheimer's Dement.* **2015**, *1*, 505–512. [CrossRef] [PubMed]

16. Meeter, L.H.; Dopper, E.G.; Jiskoot, L.C.; Sanchez-Valle, R.; Graff, C.; Benussi, L.; Ghidoni, R.; Pijnenburg, Y.A.; Borroni, B.; Galimberti, D.; et al. Neurofilament light chain: A biomarker for genetic frontotemporal dementia. *Ann. Clin. Transl. Neurol.* **2016**, *3*, 623–636. [CrossRef] [PubMed]

17. Almeida, C.G.; Takahashi, R.H.; Gouras, G.K. Beta-amyloid accumulation impairs multivesicular body sorting by inhibiting the ubiquitin-proteasome system. *J. Neurosci.* **2006**, *26*, 4277–4288. [CrossRef] [PubMed]

18. Bright, J.; Hussain, S.; Dang, V.; Wright, S.; Cooper, B.; Byun, T.; Ramos, C.; Singh, A.; Parry, G.; Stagliano, N.; et al. Human secreted tau increases amyloid-beta production. *Neurobiol. Aging* **2015**, *36*, 693–709. [CrossRef] [PubMed]

19. Kertesz, A. Rate of progression differs in frontotemporal dementia and Alzheimer disease. *Neurology* **2006**, *66*, 1607. [CrossRef] [PubMed]

20. Irimata, K.E.; Dugger, B.N.; Wilson, J.R. Impact of the Presence of Select Cardiovascular Risk Factors on Cognitive Changes among Dementia Subtypes. *Curr. Alzheimer Res.* **2018**, *15*, 1032–1044. [CrossRef] [PubMed]

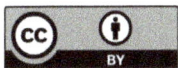

diagnostics

MDPI

Article

Functional Cognitive Disorder: Diagnostic Challenges and Future Directions

Catherine Pennington [1,2,*], Harriet Ball [1] and Marta Swirski [1]

[1]   ReMemBr Group, University of Bristol, Bristol Brain Centre, Southmead Hospital, Southmead Road, BS10 5NB Bristol, UK; harriet.ball@bristol.ac.uk (H.B.); Marta.swirski@nbt.nhs.uk (M.S.)
[2]   Centre for Dementia Prevention, University of Edinburgh, 9A Bioquarter, 9 Little France Road, Edinburgh EH16 4UX, UK
*   Correspondence: c.pennington@nhs.net

Received: 25 June 2019; Accepted: 25 September 2019; Published: 28 September 2019

Abstract: Functional cognitive disorder describes patients with persistent, troublesome subjective cognitive complaints that are inconsistent with a recognized disease process, and where significant discrepancies are found between subjective and objectively observed cognitive functioning. The etiology is heterogeneous and potentially related to underlying psychological factors. Making a diagnosis of functional cognitive disorder can be challenging and there is the potential for misdiagnosis of early-stage neurodegeneration. We compared neuropsychological findings in three groups: functional cognitive disorder (FCD), mild cognitive impairment (MCI), and healthy controls. Participants were recruited from the ReMemBr Group Clinic, North Bristol NHS Trust, and via Join Dementia Research. Both the FCD and MCI groups showed elevated prospective and retrospective memory symptom scores. Performance on the Montreal cognitive assessment was equivalent in the FCD and MCI groups, both being impaired compared with the controls. The FCD group was younger than those with MCI. We discuss challenges and controversies in the diagnosis of functional cognitive disorder, alongside illustrative cases and proposals for areas of research priority.

Keywords: functional cognitive disorder; neurodegeneration; mild cognitive impairment; functional neurological disorder cognition

1. Introduction

Functional cognitive disorder (FCD) describes patients presenting with significant subjective cognitive symptoms that are out of keeping with their observed level of cognitive functioning and not compatible with a recognizable neurodegenerative, psychiatric, or systemic primary cause [1]. In order to make a diagnosis of FCD, a marked discrepancy between self-reported cognitive symptomatology and observed or reported cognitive functioning must be present. This internal inconsistency in symptoms is evident on comparison of symptom severity with performance on neuropsychological testing or everyday "real world' cognitive ability. For example, above average performance on list learning tasks, or continued work in a skilled profession without difficulty, is inconsistent with a self-report of complete inability to recall any new information over a short time period. The etiology is heterogeneous and likely to be related to underlying psychological factors. FCD is a relatively recently described clinical entity and exists within an expanding spectrum of cognitive diagnoses, which range in severity from subjective cognitive decline (SCD) through to severe dementia. FCD is distinguished from SCD by the presence of significant inconsistency between subjective and objectively observed cognitive functioning, a greater severity of self-reported symptomatology, and resistance to reassurance that observed cognitive functioning is intact. Diagnosing FCD currently relies on expert opinion from a specialist in cognitive disorders. The optimal diagnostic criteria and management strategies for FCD are still areas of debate, and longitudinal studies of prognosis and rate of diagnostic change are lacking. Particular areas of interest are the potential for misdiagnosis of early-stage neurodegeneration, or multifactorial cognitive impairment. The prevalence of FCD is still under investigation and will vary depending on the population being studied. A review of patients attending a tertiary referral cognitive disorders clinic found a third of those aged 60 years or less to have a functional diagnosis [2]. SCD is extremely common, particularly in aging populations. A German LIFE study found that 53% of adults aged 40–79 years reported subjective memory concerns [3], whilst a USA survey identified cognitive concerns in 11.1% of adults over 45 years [4]. The SCD literature has suffered from variable terminology and definitions, which makes estimating true prevalence and incidence difficult.

Some individuals may manifest cognitive symptomatology due to a combination of etiological factors, corresponding to the concept of "functional overlay" seen in systematic and functional neurological conditions, whereby core symptoms caused by an underlying structural disease process are complicated by additional functional features [5]. A dual diagnosis of both epilepsy and psychogenic nonepileptic seizures is not uncommon [6], and individuals with chronic conditions such as multiple sclerosis may manifest additional functional symptoms, which can be misattributed [7]. In the context of cognitive symptoms, there are significant challenges around confirming diagnosis, potential for diagnostic evolution over time, and overlapping conditions. In a clinical setting, rapid access to detailed neuropsychological testing (including effort testing) is often limited, as is the use of CSF biomarkers and advanced imaging techniques, such as amyloid PET. Therefore, the distinction between neurodegenerative and functional or alternative causes for cognitive symptoms frequently depends on a combination of self-report, collateral history, and clinician opinion. The picture is further complicated by memory complaints being a common experience for healthy older adults, and psychiatric symptoms potentially being an early feature of neurodegenerative disease [8]. Therefore, careful exploration of symptom severity, evaluation of discrepancies between self-reported and observed cognitive ability, consideration of potential contributing psychological factors, beliefs or mental health symptoms, and search for evidence of neurodegenerative, toxic, or metabolic causes of cognitive decline are required when considering a diagnosis of FCD. Additionally, a correct diagnosis of FCD does not mean an individual is immune from developing future neurodegeneration.

Here, we discuss issues around prognosis, misdiagnosis, and functional overlay symptoms in FCD. We report data and illustrative cases from a recent study of FCD and MCI patients drawn from a specialist cognitive clinic.

2. Methods

Participants with FCD or MCI were recruited from a specialist cognitive disorders clinic (ReMemBr Group, North Bristol Trust). Diagnoses were reached after clinical assessment by a consultant neurologist and clinically appropriate neuroimaging and neuropsychological assessment. The diagnoses of participants recruited from the clinic were reviewed at a multidisciplinary meeting comprising three cognitive neurologists and a consultant neuropsychologist. One patient in the FCD group did not attend for subsequent clinical follow-up, and one MCI participant was recruited from Join Dementia Research. All other FCD and MCI participants attended for additional clinical follow-up in the cognitive disorders clinic.

A diagnosis of FCD was made in patients displaying significant discrepancies between self-reported and observed cognitive functioning (on neuropsychological assessment and/or everyday functioning). Exclusion criteria were evidence of neurodegeneration, toxic or metabolic causes of cognitive decline, major psychiatric disorder, or active systemic disease that could impact cognition.

Diagnoses of MCI were made based on a clinical history of mild cognitive symptoms, consisting of preserved everyday cognitive functioning and mildly impaired performance on neuropsychological testing. Only patients with MCI felt to have a neurodegenerative cause (based on investigation findings and clinical history) were included in the present study. People with toxic or metabolic causes of cognitive decline, major psychiatric disorder, or significant systemic disease that could impact cognition were excluded from this group. One additional participant with MCI was recruited from the

Join Dementia Research database; their case notes were reviewed by a cognitive neurologist (C.P.) to confirm the diagnosis. Healthy controls (HC) were recruited from a local database of adult research volunteers and the Join Dementia Research database. Controls self-identified as having no significant cognitive complaints. We did not exclude persons with mild mood or anxiety symptoms that (in the opinion of the cognitive neurology team) would not be expected to impact cognition.

Participants underwent neuropsychological testing, and demographic data were collected. This included the Montreal Cognitive Assessment (MoCA) [9], the Test of Premorbid Functioning—UK version (ToPF) [10], and the Prospective and Retrospective Memory Questionnaire (PRMQ) [11]. The MoCA is a 30-point brief cognitive assessment, with one further bonus point awarded to adults with formal education of 12 years or less. The PRMQ is a brief questionnaire asking respondents to answer 16 questions about minor everyday memory errors, using a 5-point Likert scale (from "never" to "very often"). Half of the questions refer to prospective memory, and half to retrospective. The responses are assigned values from 5 for "very often" to 1 for "never" and summed, and total scores are a minimum of 16 and maximum of 80. The ToPF provides an estimate of premorbid IQ, based on knowledge of the pronunciation of irregularly spelt words. Subjects are asked to read words with irregular grapheme–phoneme association aloud from a stimulus card. The words increase in difficulty, and the task is finished and a score assigned when errors in pronunciation occur.

The project was given Research Ethics Committee approval by the South West—Cornwall and Plymouth Research Ethics Committee, REC reference 15/SW/0298 and IRAS project ID: 188539. All participants provided informed consent. The study was funded by the BRACE charity.

Statistical analysis was undertaken using IBM SPSS Statistics version 22 and Stata version 15.1. Group comparisons were undertaken using 1-way ANOVA, or alternative tests where data did not meet assumptions for parametric data.

3. Results

A total of 21 people with FCD, 17 with MCI, and 25 HC participated in the main study. In the FCD group, all but two participants had structural neuroimaging (CT, MRI, or both). In the MCI group, all the participants had structural imaging, and six had additional functional imaging (HMPAO SPECT or DAT). The group demographics are shown in Table 1, and analysis of group differences on the PRMQ are shown in Table 2.

Table 1. Group demographics and cognitive functioning (mean values; significant *p* values in bold).

	FCD	MCI	HC	FCD vs. HC *p* Value	FCD vs. MCI *p* Value	MCI vs. HC *p* Value
Female:Male	10:11	8:9	18:7		0.15*	
Age (years)	58.3	72.1	60.8	0.30	**<0.01**	**<0.01**
Years of Education	13.8	14.4	14.7		0.61 *	
MoCA	23.9	23.3	27.8	**<0.01**	0.52	**<0.01**
ToPF	46.5	55.1	57.2	**<0.01**	**0.04**	0.87

* No significant difference across samples found; therefore, multiple comparisons not performed. Gender: Pearson's Chi-square = 3.7, *p* = 0.15; Age: Kruskal-Wallis test. Chi-square = 12.7, df = 2, *p* < 0.01; Years of education: one-way ANOVA. F = 0.5, df = 60, 2, *p* = 0.61; MoCA: Kruskal–Wallis test. Chi-square = 19.0, df = 2, *p* < 0.01; ToPF: Kruskal–Wallis test. Chi-square = 7.6, df =2, *p* = 0.02.

3.1. Case Studies

An additional two patients were recruited into the study and completed informed consent and study procedures. A subsequent case review was performed on study completion, and diagnostic uncertainty was raised in both cases. They are presented separately from the main study cohort, to illustrate potential diagnostic difficulties and change in the cognitive clinic population.

Table 2. Mean scores on the Prospective and Retrospective Memory Questionnaire.

	FCD	MCI	HC	FCD vs. HC *p* Value	FCD vs. MCI *p* Value	MCI vs. HC *p* Value
Prospective memory (raw score)	29.2	27.6	18.6	**<0.01**	0.72	**<0.01**
Retrospective memory (raw score)	25.2	25.4	16.4	**<0.01**	1.00	**<0.01**
Total T score (Prospective + Retrospective)	33.3	35.1	54.7			

Higher raw scores indicate greater self-reported memory symptoms. Lower T scores indicate greater symptomatology. T scores have a mean of 50 and SD of 10; therefore, both FCD and MCI were both approximately 2 SD below population norms. T scores were obtained using tables in Crawford et al. 2003 (Crawford et al., 2003). Analyses were repeated as an ANCOVA (controlling for age), obtaining consistent results. One-way ANOVA with Tukey post-hoc comparisons. Prospective memory raw score, F (2,60) = 19.91, $p < 0.01$. Effect size η^2 0.40 Retrospective memory raw score, F (2,60) =16.5, $p < 0.01$. Effect size η^2 0.35.

3.1.1. Case 1

A person in their sixties presented following several years of behavioral and cognitive changes. Symptom onset began around the time of a job change and an uncomplicated elective operation with subsequent opiate prescription. There was no evidence of excessive or dependent opiate use, and cognitive symptoms did not remit on the gradual cessation of opiates. The individual was less able to manage a complex occupation and had reduced empathy and extraversion. Episodic word finding difficulties were reported, exacerbated by fatigue. Symptoms improved during holiday periods.

Examination was notable for mild extrapyramidal signs. HMPAO SPECT showed frontal hypoperfusion. Negative investigations included blood tests for genetic and autoimmune causes of neurodegeneration.

On neuropsychological testing, the participant passed tests of performance validity. Most scores were in the average range, and a minority of subsets were in the low-average range. On subjective questionnaires, memory was self-rated as good, whereas their spouse rated it as significantly impaired. Depression, anxiety, and stress self-report scores were in the average range. An initial diagnosis of MCI was made.

On follow-up, MoCA scores showed an improving pattern (Figure 1). Neuropsychological testing was repeated after a one-year interval, and during this assessment, anxiety was evident. The patient also showed catastrophic interpretation of normal memory lapses. Cognitive performance results were stable or improved. A neuropsychiatric opinion highlighted exaggerated interpretation of normal memory lapses, and a revised diagnosis was made of SCD, and possible functional overlay. The individual remains under follow-up, and the trajectory of improved neuropsychology now points away from neurodegenerative processes.

3.1.2. Case 2

A person in their fifties was referred for investigation of cognitive symptoms and extensive vascular change on MRI of the brain. Two years earlier, the individual had experienced a critical illness requiring ITU stay. Following this, they had initially been able to return to previous employment but reported cognitive slowing, word-finding difficulties, and problems remembering appointments. These symptoms and stress resulted in a subsequent decision to cease work. The individual reported lack of motivation, depression and anxiety, and progressive cognitive symptoms. Their partner felt that the cognitive symptoms had been static since ceasing work. The clinical picture was complicated by poor sleep, chronic pain and opiate use, and alcohol intake. They were a current cigarette smoker, had a family history of cardiovascular disease in a first-degree relative, and dementia in second-degree relatives.

Neurological examination demonstrated jerky saccadic movements, limb weakness related to previous surgery, and chronic pain. There were no pyramidal or extrapyramidal signs. A brain MRI showed small vessel ischemic change out of proportion to age, which showed mild progression on follow-up imaging a year later. Blood tests for vasculitis and inflammatory conditions (including CADASIL genetics) were unrevealing.

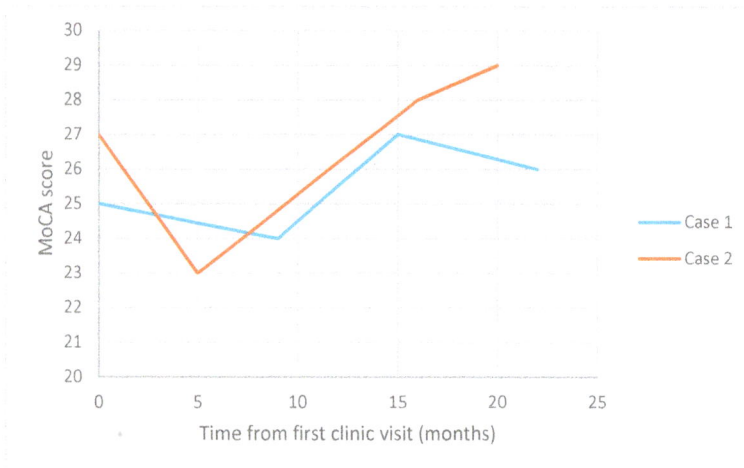

Figure 1. Serial Montreal Cognitive Assessment (MoCA) scores (bonus point included if appropriate) for illustrative cases one and two.

On neuropsychological testing, they passed tests of performance validity. Scores were low average or borderline impaired on several subsets (in particular, on word list recall, alongside average performance on short story recall). Depression and anxiety screening questionnaire scores were elevated. There were inconsistencies between self-reports of progressive cognitive symptoms in the absence of evidence of progressive cognitive decline on clinical review, and the collateral history of cognitive stability. Significant contributing adverse psychological factors were present that were felt to be impacting cognition, in conjunction with toxic and metabolic factors and vascular disease. A diagnosis of multifactorial MCI was ultimately made, and management included optimizing vascular risk factors, referral for psychological therapies, and support to attempt to reduce opiate use.

4. Discussion

In this case series of adults with FCD and neurodegenerative MCI, we found those with FCD to report an equivalent burden of cognitive symptomatology to people with MCI. Total PRMQ T scores were 33.3 in the FCD group and 35.1 in the MCI group, approximately 1.6 SD below the normative population mean [11]. This finding is in line with previous literature on functional neurological disorder, where self-ratings of disability by patients with functional symptoms are as severe or worse than those with organic neurological disease [12]. Performance on the MoCA was also indistinguishable between FCD and MCI, as both groups showed significantly impaired scores compared with the controls.

The FCD group showed lower performance on the ToPF, compared with the controls and the MCI group. The ToPF is designed to estimate premorbid cognitive abilities but is known to potentially be vulnerable to the impact of neurodegeneration and nonorganic underperformance [13]. Martin et al. examined links between performance validity test results and the ToPF, finding those failing validity tests were more likely to have a lower ToPF score than demographically predicted. People with FCD frequently show an invalid pattern of performance on neuropsychological testing [2], and it is possible that the ToPF results in the present FCD group may not accurately reflect their true premorbid baseline.

Limitations of this study include a lack of "gold standard" diagnostic criteria for FCD. Diagnostic criteria are still in evolution, and clinician judgement remains the mainstay of diagnosis. The ReMemBr Group cognitive clinic receives complex referrals from primary and secondary care; therefore, there is likely to be referral bias towards less straightforward diagnostic scenarios, which may have influenced the nature of the participants recruited in the present study. A common problem across cognitive research is a tendency for research participants to be of above population norm levels of education and socioeconomic status. Therefore, we would not consider our study sample to be truly representative of the local population, and it is possible that significant cultural differences may impact how FCD manifests and is diagnosed. Larger studies of more diverse populations in different world regions are needed to further our understanding of FCD.

Cognitive disorders are traditionally thought to reflect a binary, unidirectional process. They are present or absent, progress along a trajectory of increasing severity, and with the exception of rare, treatable causes of cognitive decline, they do not remit. This very linear view of cognition is increasingly at odds with evidence from large studies of populations with MCI, where a significant percentage of affected individuals revert to normal or near-normal cognition over time [14]. Those who improve retain an increased future risk of MCI or dementia compared to those who have not previously been diagnosed with MCI, and thus, they may move between diagnostic categories more than once during their cognitive journey [15,16]. Individuals with SCD are also highly heterogeneous. The SCIENCe cohort study subdivided people with SCD into those with preclinical Alzheimer's disease (AD; based on CSF or PET amyloid positivity), those with very mild psychiatric symptoms, and the remainder of individuals with features of neither [17]. A classification of preclinical AD was associated with older age and Apolipoprotein E4 status. Those with psychiatric features reported a greater degree of cognitive symptomatology than those with preclinical AD. Other studies of the long-term prognosis of SCD have identified a variety of potential clinical trajectories, including symptom remittance. Those with persistent symptoms reported over a number of time points appear to be at greater risk of progression to MCI or dementia, whilst those who intermittently report cognitive symptoms are not at increased risk, compared to people who have never reported cognitive symptoms [18]. Clearly, in the instances of SCD and MCI, diagnostic status is often a dynamic concept.

Our case reports highlight the potential for cognitive multimorbidity and diagnostic change over time. Case 1 was initially diagnosed with MCI, but this was revised on clinical follow up to SCD, with a possible element of functional overlay. Potential "red flags" for future cognitive decline are present in this case, based on the abnormal HMPAO SPECT, and cognitive changes being noted by close informants. Symptoms reported by significant others is regarded as a pointer towards neurodegeneration, as opposed to self-reported symptoms [19]. Contrarily, the improvement in MoCA performance would go against a neurodegenerative process, and the observed tendency to catastrophic thinking is a positive feature of functional symptoms. Given the diagnostic ambiguity, it could be argued that this patient might benefit from advanced neurodegenerative biomarker analysis with amyloid or tau imaging, and CSF analysis. However, these tests are not yet widely available in the UK NHS, and there is potential for iatrogenic harm by over-investigation, either through physical complications or adverse psychological consequences.

The diagnosis of FCD depends on expert clinician opinion, with the use of targeted clinical investigations. The clinical picture in FCD is of a significant burden of persistent cognitive symptoms, which cause patient distress and worry, but objective cognitive deficits are inconsistent with self-reported symptoms—this may be based on neuropsychological assessment, or self or collateral reports of activities requiring a high level of cognitive functioning. The discrepancy between symptoms and behavior is key to the diagnosis of FCD, and additional positive features are resistance to reassurance, repeated medical consultations, and failure of performance validity tests.

Case 2 illustrates the multifactorial nature of cognitive changes experienced by many patients, and the potential for functional symptoms to overlay other cognitive pathologies. The patient had been exposed to significant serious systemic morbidity, had evidence of neuronal injury on neuroimaging, in addition to ongoing issues with psychoactive medications, alcohol, and sleep pathology. There were also significant mental health symptoms, and the clinical impression was of functional symptoms contributing to the cognitive picture. It is extremely challenging to unpick the contributions of these different factors. A pragmatic management strategy should aim to improve potentially reversible factors, such as sleep, mental health, and cognitive toxin intake. Longitudinal follow-up is often needed, as the pattern of cognitive change (or lack thereof) is of diagnostic value, particularly to avoid missing neurodegeneration in complex individuals. The possibility of mental health symptoms arising as part of a dementia prodrome should be considered, particularly in older adults and those without a past history of mental health disorders.

Findings from our case series comparison of groups with FCD, MCI, and healthy controls show that PRMQ scores were equivalent in both the FCD and MCI groups, as was MoCA performance. This is despite expert opinion that those in the FCD group reported cognitive symptoms that were disproportionate to their observed cognitive functioning. Therefore, the PRMQ may not capture sufficiently detailed self-reported symptoms to be used diagnostically. The presence of a major discrepancy between subjective and objective cognition remains the mainstay of FCD diagnosis. More detailed exploration of neuropsychological features of FCD is warranted to seek out potential condition specific features that can aid in diagnosis. The potential for a diagnosis of FCD to change over time has not yet been explored, and there are little data available on the long-term prognosis. The optimal extent of investigations and follow-up is also unresolved. A deep phenotyping study of FCD will shortly open at the University of Edinburgh [20]. It is hoped that this and other future studies will establish clear diagnostic criteria for FCD and provide insight into causative mechanisms and avenues for potential therapeutic developments. Clinicians and researchers should be mindful of the potential for both diagnostic overlap and diagnostic change over time.

Author Contributions: C.P.—study design, data analysis, manuscript writing and editing; H.B.—data analysis and manuscript editing; M.S.—participant recruitment and evaluation.

Funding: The study was funded by a project grant from the BRACE charity.

Acknowledgments: We would like to thank all the study participants for their support of this work. Additionally, we would like to acknowledge recruitment support from the Join Dementia Research platform. Join Dementia Research is funded by the Department of Health and delivered by the National Institute for Health Research in partnership with Alzheimer Scotland, Alzheimer's Research UK and Alzheimer's Society.

Conflicts of Interest: The authors have no conflict of interest to declare.

References

1. Pennington, C.; Hayre, A.; Newson, M.; Coulthard, E. Functional Cognitive Disorder: A Common Cause of Subjective Cognitive Symptoms. *J. Alzheimer's Dis.* **2015**, *48*, S19–S24. [CrossRef] [PubMed]

2. Stone, J.; Pal, S.; Blackburn, D.; Reuber, M.; Thekkumpurath, P.; Carson, A. Functional (Psychogenic) Cognitive Disorders: A Perspective from the Neurology Clinic. *J. Alzheimer's Dis.* **2015**, *49*, S5–S17. [CrossRef] [PubMed]

3. Luck, T.; Roehr, S.; Rodriguez, F.S.; Schroeter, M.L.; Witte, A.V.; Hinz, A.; Mehner, A.; Engel, C.; Loeffler, M.; Thiery, J.; et al. Memory-related subjective cognitive symptoms in the adult population: Prevalence and associated factors - results of the LIFE-Adult-Study. *BMC Psychol.* **2018**, *21*, 6. [CrossRef] [PubMed]

4. Taylor, C.A.; Bouldin, E.D.; McGuire, L.C. Subjective cognitive decline among adults aged ≥45 years—United States, 2015–2016. *Morb. Mortal. Wkly. Rep.* **2018**, *67*, 754–757. [CrossRef] [PubMed]

5. Stone, J.; Reuber, M.; Carson, A. Functional symptoms in neurology: Mimics and chameleons. *Pract. Neurol.* **2013**, *13*, 104–113. [CrossRef] [PubMed]

6. Kutlubaev, M.A.; Xu, Y.; Hackett, M.L.; Stone, J. Dual diagnosis of epilepsy and psychogenic nonepileptic seizures: Systematic review and meta-analysis of frequency, correlates, and outcomes. *Epilepsy Behav.* **2018**, *89*, 70–78. [CrossRef] [PubMed]

7. Merwick, A.; Sweeney, B. Functional symptoms in clinically definite MS–pseudo-relapse syndrome. *Int. MS J.* **2008**, *15*, 47–51. [PubMed]

8. Stella, F.; Radanovic, M.; Balthazar, M.L.F.; Canineu, P.R.; De Souza, L.C.; Forlenza, O.V. Neuropsychiatric Symptoms in the Prodromal Stages of Dementia. *Curr. Opin. Psychiatry.* **2014**, *27*, 230–235. [CrossRef] [PubMed]

9. Nasreddine, Z.S.; Phillips, N.A.; Bédirian, V.; Charbonneau, S.; Whitehead, V.; Collin, I.; Cummings, J.; Certkow, H. The Montreal Cognitive Assessment, MoCA: A brief screening tool for mild cognitive impairment. *J. Am. Geriatr. Soc.* **2005**, *53*, 695–699. [CrossRef] [PubMed]

10. Pearson. Test of Premorbid Functioning, UK Version. Administration, Scoring and Techniques Manual. Available online: https://www.pearsonclinical.co.uk/Psychology/AdultCognitionNeuropsychologyandLanguage/AdultGeneralAbilities/TOPF/TestofPremorbidFunctioning.aspx (accessed on 20 September 2019).

11. Crawford, J.R.; Smith, G.; Maylor E a Della Sala, S.; Logie, R.H. The Prospective and Retrospective Memory Questionnaire (PRMQ): Normative data and latent structure in a large non-clinical sample. *Memory* **2003**, *11*, 261–275. [CrossRef] [PubMed]

12. Carson, A.; Stone, J.; Hibberd, C.; Murray, G.; Duncan, R.; Coleman, R.; Warlow, C.; Roberts, R.; Pelosi, A.; Cavanagh, J.; et al. Disability, distress and unemployment in neurology outpatients with symptoms "unexplained by organic disease". *J. Neurol. Neurosurg. Psychiatry* **2011**, *82*, 810–813. [CrossRef] [PubMed]

13. Martin, P.K.; Schroeder, R.W.; Wyman-Chick, K.A.; Hunter, B.P.; Heinrichs, R.J.; Baade, L.E. Rates of Abnormally Low TOPF Word Reading Scores in Individuals Failing Versus Passing Performance Validity Testing. *Assessment* **2018**, *25*, 640–652. [CrossRef] [PubMed]

14. Ganguli, M.; Jia, Y.; Hughes, T.F.; Snitz, B.E.; Chang, C.C.H.; Berman, S.B.; Sullivan KIlyas Kamboh, M. Mild Cognitive Impairment that Does Not Progress to Dementia: A Population-Based Study. *J. Am. Geriatr. Soc.* **2019**, *67*, 232–238. [CrossRef] [PubMed]

15. Aerts, L.; Heffernan, M.; Kochan, N.A.; Crawford, J.D.; Draper, B.; Trollor, J.N.; Brodaty, H. Effects of MCI subtype and reversion on progression to dementia in a community sample. *Neurology* **2017**, *88*, 2225–2232. [CrossRef] [PubMed]

16. Koepsell, T.D.; Monsell, S.E. Reversion from mild cognitive impairment to normal or near-Normal cognition; Risk factors and prognosis. *Neurology* **2012**, *79*, 1591–1598. [CrossRef] [PubMed]

17. Slot, R.E.R.; Verfaillie, S.C.J.; Overbeek, J.M.; Timmers, T.; Wesselman, L.M.P.; Teunissen, C.E.; Bols, A.; Bouwman, F.; Prins, N.; Barkhof, F.; et al. Subjective Cognitive Impairment Cohort (SCIENCe): Study design and first results. *Alzheimer's Res. Ther.* **2018**, *10*, 1–13. [CrossRef] [PubMed]

18. Roehr, S.; Villringer, A.; Angermeyer, M.C.; Luck, T.; Riedel-Heller, S.G. Outcomes of stable and unstable patterns of subjective cognitive decline—Results from the Leipzig Longitudinal Study of the Aged (LEILA75+). *BMC Geriatr.* **2016**, *16*, 1–8. [CrossRef] [PubMed]

19. Valech, N.; Mollica, M.A.; Olives, J.; Tort, A.; Fortea, J.; Lleo, A.; Belen, S.; Molinuevo, J.; Rami, L. Informant's Perception of Subjective Cognitive Decline Helps to Discriminate Preclinical Alzheimer's Disease from Normal Aging. *J. Alzheimer's Dis.* **2015**, *48*, S87–S98. [CrossRef] [PubMed]

20. McWhirter, L.; Ritchie, C.W.; Carson, A.J.; Stone, J. Improving Diagnosis in Cognitive Disorders. 2019. Available online: https://www.protocols.io/view/improving-diagnosis-in-cognitive-disorders-z97f99n/abstract (accessed on 28 September 2019).

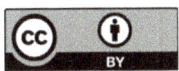

MDPI

St. Alban-Anlage 66

4052 Basel

Switzerland

Tel. +41 61 683 77 34

Fax +41 61 302 89 18

www.mdpi.com

Diagnostics Editorial Office

E-mail: diagnostics@mdpi.com

www.mdpi.com/journal/diagnostics

www.ingramcontent.com/pod-product-compliance
Lightning Source LLC
Chambersburg PA
CBHW051909210326
41597CB00033B/6085